Bow Ti
Butterflies
&
Band-Aids

A journey through
childhood cancers
and back to life

Lindsey VanDyke

ISBN: 145053564X
ISBN-13: 9781450535649
LCCN: 2010900927

O f all the cancer/survivor biographies out there, many are written by celebrities. Few are about the process of growing up with cancer. I saw a need for a definitive description of feelings, perceptions, and fears as I saw them—through the eyes of a child who was in the process of morphing into an adult. When I was going through treatment, I was always afraid, but more afraid to talk about it because I didn't want people to laugh at me or think I was stupid. Part of me feared what answers I might get. I had enough on my plate just getting through the day, thank you very much.

This story is, to the best of my memories, an accurate depiction of my life with cancer from the 'tweens through young adulthood. I also enlisted the memories of those who have been close to me and who could shed light on some events that are no longer clear in my mind. I have done my best to reconstruct conversations as my friends and family and I remember them. In the interest of privacy, some names have been changed.

My intent for this work is to provide some insight and companionship to patients, parents, siblings, and friends when their worlds have been flipped upside down. I hope that when kids read about my elaborately contrived fears, they can say, "Whew! I'm not the only one," and when they read about my additional anxieties about dating and peer acceptance, they have something to relate to when no one else can relate with them. I hope that caregivers can understand more of what might be going through their patient's head as the table slides into the MRI machine, or as they send their patients off out into the world when they reach their cure date. When parents read this, I hope they can be relieved to understand more about what their child might be experiencing from his or her point of view, and open better dialogue between them. If my story provides comfort or inspiration to only one reader, then I did my job correctly.

For mom.

For Wolff.

For all the families just starting

their cancer journey today.

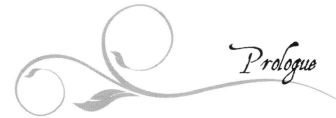

I stared up at the ceiling into the soft, greenish glow of the fluorescent lights, wondering if I would have time to count all the little dots in the acoustic ceiling tiles. *They sure are taking their sweet time*, I thought. As the minutes ticked by my mind wandered, pondering the gravity of what was about to happen to me. I'd never had surgery before. Suddenly, it hit me. *M*A*S*H*. I'd just seen it a couple weeks ago: the episode where the supply lines had been cut, and they were running out of anesthesia, so they had to lower everyone's doses. One guy *woke up in the middle of surgery*. Oh. My. *God*. What if they ran out of anesthesia in the middle of *my* surgery? How were we supposed to know if the anesthesia man made his delivery this morning?

As my hysteria over this completely irrational thought built, Mom and Dad were allowed in. It looked as though I had been bumped for an emergency surgery, and that's why we had been in pre-op so long. I didn't want them to think I was crazy, so I didn't mention what I had seen on *M*A*S*H* or that the same thing was totally going to happen today. Because, you know. The Korean War front lines are *exactly* the same as a prestigious hospital in Portland, Oregon, in 1991.

The three of us chatted about various things while we waited, but much of the time was spent in silent anticipation, wondering how we all ended up here. In the last seventy-two hours our lives made a total 180. I'd become very ill very quickly, and here we were in Doernbecher Children's Hospital awaiting confirmation of what my new team of doctors suspected was a very advanced cancer.

After a while, a pack of white-coats entered our curtained cubicle. *They always travel in packs*, I thought. Later I found out why: one or two of them were teachers, and the rest were still in training. This hospital was a school, but it didn't look anything like any school I'd ever seen. A middle-aged man, who introduced himself as Dr. Henricks, was in charge. "Do you have any questions?" he asked. I shook my head. "All right then. It'll be about ten minutes while we all go get ready, OK?"

"OK." Seriously. What was I supposed to say? No, it's not OK. If you please, I'd rather just go home now and pretend none of this has happened. Yeah. That would fly with Mama Linda.

My mom disappeared for a while, asking the doctor some questions. It was just Dad and me. I was becoming increasingly internally restless. Finally, I could stand it no longer. My one irrational fear had snowballed.

"Dad! What if they run out of anesthesia while I'm in there?"

He looked at me blandly, either shocked by my stupidity or afraid that I was thinking too hard about it. I hoped it was the latter. "They won't run out."

"But I saw it on *M*A*S*H*! They ran out, and this guy *woke up* in the middle and started screaming!"

"That's just a TV show; it's not real. Besides, this is the best kids' hospital in Oregon, not a mobile army hospital in the Korean War. They don't ever let that kind of thing happen in real life."

"But what if the power goes out or something? And all the lights go out and they can't see what they're doing?"

"It won't happen. I'm sure they have backup generators just in case."

"OK." I thought for a minute, trying to cover all the horrible possibilities. "But what if there's an earthquake or something?"

"There won't be an earthquake. Even if there *was* one, this building is probably the safest in the whole city. It's built very, very strong."

I didn't have time to query further. Someone was back to get me. I couldn't tell if it was one of the white-coats I'd seen before or someone else. He—or she—had a mask on and one of those puffy paper hairnets. It made me think of a mushroom. Mom had returned, too, and so away we went, me on the gurney, Mom and Dad walking next to me. When we got to the double doors marked, "Sterile Area: Authorized Hospital Personnel Only," Dad squeezed my hands and said,

"We'll see you when you're out. Just count back from one hundred and it'll be over in no time." Mom kissed me on the head as I rolled through the automatic double doors into surgery and out of childhood.

PART ONE:
The Cancer

A ll things considered, I had a pretty sweet childhood. I was given almost anything I wanted. We didn't live in a big house or take big exotic vacations every summer like some of our friends did, but Mom and Dad scraped up the money every year to put my brother and me through private school, and that was worth sacrificing yearly vacations.

My parents are *Green Acres*. My mother, Linda, born and raised in suburbia, is a powerful woman who loves bronzer, coral lipsticks, and big jewelry. The paragon of micromanaging, she's a talker and a Type A all the way. Her profession dictated that everything and everyone look just so, and those traits also carried over into our home life. She drives a Mercedes that's as big as her personality. Mama Linda is always in charge. And she can *always* be depended upon. Conversely, my father, Wes, is her opposite: born and raised on a farm, he prefers quiet observation away from people and is never interested in standing out, making a statement, or for that matter, looking "just so." In contrast to her fashionable flair, you would most likely see him in an old T-shirt, Levis 501s discolored by years of grease and dirt, a pair of old Nikes that have seen better days, and a baseball cap brandishing the logo for a local grain elevator, seed company, or farm implement. In the summer his face and arms darken so much from working outdoors that he looks almost Latino, but underneath that shirt and those jeans, he's the poster-child for the whitey-white Dutch race everywhere. Up until 1999, he still drove his first car: a 1966 red GMC pickup which at any given time could be found in varying states of disrepair that had forced him to replace the bed, floorboards, most of the engine, and the paint.

Juxtaposed, my parents are an unlikely pair but nonetheless a very balanced combination. Mom owns and operates her own interior design business, and Dad operates the farm established by his father, which is now shared among his many siblings. We lived in Cornelius, a rural town outside of Portland, Oregon. In those days the population was only a few thousand, and today most of what I remember as strawberry fields and cow pastures is, sadly, now subdivisions and pavement. Even the most rural areas are not lonely today as they were when I was a kid. I remember my days roaming freely around the farm, accompanied only by our dogs Sassy and Sandy Dunes, or often just alone. I never wondered if transients were hiding in our property or if there were used needles lying around. Maybe I should have. I would roam the property at will and walk alone under the big bridge and throw stones into the Tualatin River where it swooshed over a small ridge of rocks. I'd crawl down the banks near where Dad would install the irrigation pumps every spring and watch the eddy swirl endlessly, entrapping fallen leaves, and see the crayfish scoot along the muddy bottom. Today, the crawdads are dead from chemical runoff from the nurseries upstream, and there is evidence all over that there are others on our place.

Our place consisted of about fifty acres. In the wintertime, most of it would flood when the Tualatin swelled over its banks. We would have lakefront property for a few months, and Dad would take me and my brother Travis out in the boat. Travis was five years my junior, and hell on wheels. He once told our principal, Sister Mary, to "hasta la vista, baby" when he was in the 2nd grade. We often didn't get along back then, but then what brother/sister combination does? We had our moments of unity, though, like when dad was piloting our little boat across the floodwaters. We always squealed happily when he could get the small aluminum boat to catch air over its wakes.

Our house was perched above the flood plain on a small hill. We lived in a square yellow house with blue shutters and two small landings for our front and back porches. We got our water from the original well, so there was a small pump house in the back yard that housed, well, the well pump. We had a pet goat, Zucchini, tethered to a long run in front of his A-frame chalet just beyond the back yard. He kept the thistles and briar bushes down, and acted on the side as a garbage disposal—his favorite snack by far was moldy bread. A few times he snapped his tie, and he'd go straight for one of the porches and poop on it. Every time. If it was a hot day and the doors were open, he might march straight through the screen, and Mom would chase him back out of the house, cursing under her breath.

There was an apple orchard, and in our front yard were a pair of oak trees that were saplings when Abraham Lincoln was president. Two walnut trees shaded the long gravel driveway that bisected a large field. After a rainfall, you could walk through the fields and find arrowheads and other artifacts left over from when local Native Americans inhabited the Tualatin River basin, or bits of broken pottery from families who lived there long before us. I once found the porcelain torso of a doll that lacked, like classic European sculptures, a head and arms.

Almost every day, I'd cross the road to Grandma and Papa's place. Once, as a toddler, I'd done it without my mother's knowledge and was strongly admonished from doing that ever again. The next time, I just walked down underneath the bridge and back up to the farmhouse. Because I never actually crossed the road again, Mom and Dad were a little confused as to whether I deserved punishment.

Grandma and Papa still lived on the original farm, about eighty acres. Though well into retirement, they still had plenty of animals on site. I'd chase the chickens, find their nests, and smash the eggs on the wall of the steer pen for sport. I'd feed the pigs or try to pet the steers (who always ran away—it seems they knew what was to become of them). In the yard, Papa grew grapes, which became wine. There were always bird coops where the hens were laying, and plenty of warm, fuzzy yellow chicks. The hens would puff up and emit deep warning clucks if you got to close to their brood.

Once, when I was very young, I picked up a chick to pet it, and the hen flew on my head and pecked me until I put it back. I was careful after that, and my forehead still shows a pockmark.

Farming is always at odds with nature. For example, there were times during the process of cutting hay when the crew would accidentally run a pheasant through the machine. Papa would call a halt to the whole works until they could find her nest, and someone would run the small light green-and-black speckled eggs back to the yard as quickly as possible and slide them under a nesting hen. Different animal populations suffered in different ways. Even before my lifetime, the pheasant population was in decline, and Papa firmly believed in doing his part to keep alive what farming often destroys. Foxes were another animal at risk; Papa once saved a fox cub when the vixen met the fate of the hay mower. We did our best to give back to the environment.

It really is a joy to grow up on a farm. On ours, there was no shortage of cats, kittens, dogs, puppies, chickens, pigs, cows, and pigeons. Occasionally there was a bunny in the big coop, and once we had a very ornate type of pheasant, which I dubbed "The Pretty Bird." Colorful and beautiful as it was, it had a temper—it would chase you if you got too close. When I was ten years old, I got a horse. She was an eighteen-year-old bay quarter horse named Misty with a little white star on her forehead, a crooked stripe down her slightly roman nose, and a white snip on her upper lip.

Because of my proximity to the farm, I was very close with my grandparents. If I saw Papa when I got there, he'd say, "It's the Boo!" Various family members had graced me with a number of nicknames centered around "Boo." Booie. Boo-Boo. The Boo. The Sweet Baboo. And somehow, "Bambino" grew out of that, too. I might go with Papa to hunt gophers that were eating our crops out by the roots. We'd putter down the pasture road on an old, school-bus-yellow 1952 Honda motorcycle. If the gophers weren't having a smorgasbord, the Canadian geese were, but the blast from an air gun made quick work of them. Sometimes we'd see vultures circling overhead, coyotes running on the horizon, or prints marking the passing of a cougar. Mostly, you could see where deer had bedded down, flattening the thick canary grass. In the late winter, Papa would venture into the forest looking for

Snowdrops–tiny, white, delicate flowers that he would uproot and transplant to Grandma's flowerbeds.

If I saw Grandma, she would greet me demurely, and maybe we would bake cobbler, cake, or her signature apple tart. The woman never used a recipe. The tart was made with the Gravensteins from the tree in her own yard, pie dough heavy with shortening, a scattering of cornflakes, and topped with a wash of milk, egg white, and sugar. I might help Papa kill a hen for dinner, then watch Grandma pluck and prepare the chicken or a wild duck that had been shot in one of our duck ponds. She taught me to make applesauce, jam, root beer, and canned fruit. If it was autumn, we would plant tulips. In the spring it was foxglove, snapdragons, or a vegetable garden. She showed me that coffee grounds and ashes from the wood furnace help things grow. In the summer we would pick plums or tiny apples from a miniature tree, and in the fall it was time for the fat purple grapes. In wintertime, when it was cold and rainy out, she taught me how to embroider. Suffice it to say I learned a lot from my grandma.

In the spring, Jeanna, my dad's only sister out of the eight kids, would round up all us grandkids and we'd walk down from the farmhouse to the forest in search of Trilliums. Somehow, the poison oak always managed to find Jeanna, but it was worth it when we would part two big ferns and in between lay the prize: a cluster of tiny, white, three-petal flowers on a stalk looming above three enormous green leaves. I always liked the older blooms because they turned a violent shade of purple.

My dad's family was large. He had seven siblings that all grew up on this farm–seven boys and one girl. As kids they milked cows, tended crops and lived an almost self-sustained life. For the most part, everyone still lived in the general vicinity of the farm, so holidays and other family events were always packed with aunts, uncles, and cousins. Jeanna was our favorite aunt, and with no children of her own, she became an extra mother to all of us–especially to me. She always had the most vibrant personality and the most expressive smile. Being an actress, she knew a thing or two about good storytelling and knew how to pantomime sewing her lips shut, a skill which us nieces and nephews all found thoroughly disgusting and simultaneously delightful. At holidays, she taught us song and dance routines, some of which still exist (to my chagrin) on 8 mm. She and I had a bit together singing Lee Morse's 1925 hit, "Yes Sir, That's My Baby." Time with Jeanna always meant fun. It always meant adventure.

Every fall, Dad's brothers and Papa would go hunting for venison. A steer and some pigs were slaughtered. Out of the three came our family's tradition: sausage, by a recipe that is rumored to have come to Oregon from the Old World more than a century ago. The men hand-ground, hand-packed, hand-smoked, hand-wrapped, and hand-distributed it to everyone in the family. Travis and I went to Visitation Catholic School in Washington County's Dutch-German heartland of Verboort, where there was a sausage festival every November that attracted visitors from all over the northwest. Every pound of that sausage was similarly handmade from the same recipe handed down among our family for the last century.

This was life. It was a good life. I cannot imagine having another life.

For most of my friends, however–Holly being my best friend–this was not "normal." They did not live on farms. This was "cool." But along with the family bonds and farm animals, you get a lot of exposure to life. And believe me, you learn about all life's angles on a farm. You experience birth, and you experience death. Sometimes they happen one right after the other. You learn about growing things and some of the necessities life demands in return. Every seed gets harvested. Every animal will eventually die, including us. And from time to time, in between the beginning and the end, things go impossibly wrong.

November 9, 1991, is a day that will live in infamy for me. It's hard for me to imagine that for millions of other people it was just a regular old Friday. I'm sure they were all looking forward to the weekend; maybe they were getting ready for Thanksgiving. I remember it was clear and sunny and unseasonably warm for early November.

My brother Travis's birthday party was on November 9. He and roughly a dozen or so other six-year-olds amassed at the Forest Grove Gymnastics Center for his party. I was there, too, with Holly. We trampolined, ran obstacles, swung on the rings, ate birthday cake, and ran ourselves exhausted. It was a fantastic time.

After the party was over, another of my friends, Kristin, came over to our house. We were painting pictures of horses when it happened. My stomach started to hurt very suddenly. Not nausea, but a terrible, throbbing ache. Finally, I couldn't ignore it anymore. I went to Mom and she told me to take two Tylenol. Two hours later, the pain was worse. I curled up on my bed in the fetal position. Kristin continued her work at the easel. Suddenly, I had to pee in a major way. So, I got up and walked into the bathroom. When I sat down, I felt as though something had burst. When I stood up I saw only dark, black blood in the toilet.

I freaked. "Mom! I went to the bathroom and there was a lot of blood. Like a *lot*."

She looked at me a second, her eyes wide. "Is it still there?"

"No, I flushed it."

She relaxed a little then, as though a light went off in her head. I was eleven. I had abdominal pain and there was blood in the toilet. *Of course*. So she showed me how to use a maxi pad, and I took two more Tylenol–which I hated doing because I could never swallow the pills right the first time and my reward was a nauseating bitter aftertaste. I went back into my room. Kristin looked at me and said sympathetically and knowingly, "I heard what happened. It happened to me last year. It sucks."

By five o'clock the pain was still increasing, and I had to pee again. I felt that same bursting sensation, and there was even more black blood in the toilet. Not so much as a drop on the pad. By this time, it was clear that the Tylenol wasn't working, and even I could tell that my "period" seemed to be behaving oddly. This time I didn't flush it and showed Mom, who immediately decided that Kristin should go home. I lay down on my bed again, and Mom came in. She said, "It still hurts? Let me see your stomach."

I raised the shirt and it was visible: on the left side, an enormous bulge below my ribs. She felt it; it was hard and unyielding. I don't remember what happened next, except that we drove immediately to Tuality Hospital Emergency Room.

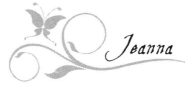

Jeanna

Linda drove over to the farm where my husband Jeff and I were for the day and said, "I'm looking for Wes, I've got to find Wes, I have to take Lindsey to the hospital." And Lindsey was sitting in the backseat, sobbing. Her hair was wet and she was wrapped in a blanket. Linda told me that she was bleeding and had a swelling in her abdomen. When Linda talked to the doctor, he'd said to come in as soon as possible. She dropped Travis off with us to take care of him.

I anxiously kept watch for Wes out the kitchen window and finally saw him drive in to the driveway with a group of guys. I went outside to talk to him. It was so awkward to me because it was getting dark and I couldn't see anyone's face. I tried to be discreet telling him what had happened in front of all these men I didn't know. I don't know if I used my mom's phrase "down there" or not, in describing the bleeding. It was weird because he'd been having a good time with his friends and didn't seem all that anxious to get out of the car. I think he was thinking, What, did she break her arm again?

He rumbled off to the hospital in his old red pickup, and I went back inside to watch Home Alone *with Travis. After awhile, Wes called to say he needed someone to come and get his truck at the hospital. I said, "OK, I'll go get Roger and we'll come." Roger is our brother. Wes said, "OK. But don't bring Travis with you. Get somebody to watch him." I said, "Well what is it?" He said in almost a whisper, "Oh, it's bad. It's bad."*

We waited for what seemed like hours before they gave me a room. I thought with that sense of entitlement that only a 'tween can have, *Don't they understand how much blood I'm peeing? Jeez, you'd think they could move a little faster.* Maybe if we'd called an ambulance I wouldn't have to wait. The pain was unbearable. When I finally went to the room, I curled up on the table. After another lengthy wait, a doctor came in and started examining me. He felt the mass, took my vitals, and decided that it was a blockage in the colon. He proceeded to do a rectal exam to confirm this diagnosis.

I endured it without protest because I figured he knew how to stop the pain. So there I was, lying on the table, thinking only about the pain and wondering how I went from the trampoline to a rectal exam so quickly.

Mom, of course, was dissatisfied. "How does that explain the bleeding?" she demanded. "I want a second opinion."

Dr. Neidermeyer was the pediatrician on call that night. He ordered some X-rays of my abdomen and asked me some questions about my urinary and bowel habits. I'd never heard the word "bowel" before, but it's one of those words that you can instinctively know. I was in agony, so much so that I found it difficult to lie straight and still for the X-ray. By the time the films were back, I was starting to get angry. *Why can't they do anything for my pain? How can they not know what's causing this? Why have we been here so long?* All I wanted was to go home to my bed. I wouldn't see my own bed for almost two weeks.

Dr. Neidermeyer showed Mom and Dad the films while a nurse inserted an IV and administered something. That was the one time in my life that an IV was quick and painless—I was too distracted by the louder pain to notice much. I don't know what they gave me that night, but I fought hard to stay awake. Next thing I knew, Aunt Jeanna was there, and so was mom's friend Sharon, whose husband is an oncologist at Tuality Hospital. I knew that her husband was an oncologist, but I didn't know what that meant. Sharon told me later that as she ran down the hallway in the ER, she saw Dad standing in the hallway crying. The image of my Dad sobbing shamelessly in public is the most horrible thing I've ever had to process in my brain. I am thankful I didn't see it myself.

Between three and six o'clock, Lindsey came to me and said she didn't feel good. By four or five o'clock, I knew something was seriously wrong. By six thirty p.m. we had a diagnosis. But one of the doctors at the ER tried to tell me that there was something else wrong. He said she probably didn't have cancer; she probably just needed an enema, and that he would do one soon. I said, "Bullshit. Until I actually see the doctor I talked to on the phone, we don't do anything."

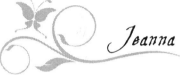

I walked through the doors to the emergency room and saw everyone standing there. I saw Linda's parents; Shirley was red faced and crying. Royal looked ashen, solemn, and would not look me in the face. I remember thinking, This is truly a bad thing. *And the weight kept getting heavier on my chest. Sharon was there. Lindsey's X-rays were on the light board. Sharon pointed to the X-ray and said, "This is what is bad" indicating the tumors. I had never seen an X-ray before, but the tumors were quite easy to point out: a really big one on the left side of her stomach and then a scattering of small tumors in her lungs.*

I was distraught. Oh my God, my little girl—the closest thing I have to a daughter—has tumors in her lungs. *Linda came out, and she was all stressed out, too. "Oh, Jeanna, she's gonna want to see you."* Oh, God. How do I do that? *I took a second to straighten out my face and walked into Lindsey's room.*

"Hi, Jeanna! How are you?" She was smiling. I was relieved; she made it so easy to be there with her. It was a relief because everyone else that night was wailing. Lindsey had no idea of what we were all up against yet. "Where's Jeff?" she asked immediately. The nurse said, "Oh, is Jeff your dog?" We laughed because Jeff is actually my husband. My mantra became "Let's Make Things Easier for Her" instead of thinking about what it was doing to me.

She looked good. It was probably because of the drugs, but she was laughing and cheerful. She just didn't look sick at all.

I got down to the ER and Dr. Neidermeyer was the pediatrician on call that night. He showed us the X-rays and showed us the spots and said that he thought it was cancer. My first thought was that it was lung cancer and that she was a goner. It hit me really, really hard. Devastated, I thought, We just as well should start making funeral plans. *After several hours and after we had gotten to OHSU and met Dr. Wolff, we found out what kind of cancer it actually probably was and that made a big difference.*

How ignorant I was. I thought it was lung cancer, not Wilms Tumor to *the lungs. It makes a world of difference. We learned later that Wilms is the most common childhood kidney cancer, and that it sends metastases to the lungs most commonly. The good news about it is that it's easily treatable and can have cure rates upwards of 80-90%, whereas true lung cancer like we see in grown-ups is often a death sentence.*

Hours passed. I faded in and out of sleep on the hard exam table. I had no idea what time it was then, but someone told me that I was going to get to ride in an ambulance and that the ambulance was taking me to the children's hospital in Portland.

"Maybe if you ask, the driver will turn on the lights for you" the nurse said, trying in vain to be cheerful. I remember the look on her face. I think she knew. I thought, *Hey, that actually might be neat to ride in an ambulance.* I also remembered Mom telling me before how cool the inside of an ambulance is, and so while I waited, I wondered about the fantastic things they must keep in there.

When it came time to go, they scooted me from the exam table to the gurney, and away we went. I was impressed at how smoothly they could collapse the gurney to go in the ambulance. I'd always had an irrational fear that I'd break my leg and be on one of those things and they wouldn't be able to collapse it. I'd lay there screaming as they shook it up and down, up and down, trying to get those wheels to accordion up. I watched too much

Rescue, 911! on TV. Mom rode in the back next to me, and Jeanna rode shotgun. Sharon and Dad tailed the ambulance.

When everyone was in, they closed the doors at my feet and we were off. I looked up at the ceiling. To my left and slightly behind me was Mom. To my right was the paramedic. Right above my head was a bag with a thin clear hose that attached to my IV Everything else was disappointing. Near my right leg was a big cabinet with what seemed like a hundred little drawers. Each was neatly labeled. Bor-ring. I can't remember most of it; I was half asleep. I could see some other plastic things on the walls—some tubing and masks—but for the most part this ambulance was not nearly as cool as everyone had made it out to be.

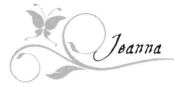

Jeanna

When it was time to transport her to Doernbecher, she wanted me to go along in place of her mom. I said, "No, your mom will go with you, and if there's room I'll go, too." There was only room for one, but the paramedics let me ride shotgun. We couldn't really talk to each other during the drive, so we hollered, "Brain thoughts! Brain thoughts!" to each other. "Brain thoughts" was our phrase that meant, "I'm thinking of you."

At one point during the drive, the ambulance driver muttered, "Doernbecher. Is that the one on the hill?" I wondered if he was talking on a radio headset. Finally, I asked, "Are you talking to me?" "Yeah," he said. "Is Doernbecher the hospital on the hill?" I exclaimed, "How am I supposed to know?"

It took about a half hour to make it to the hill where the Oregon Health and Science University Hospital and Doernbecher Children's Hospital are. I kept trying to make myself ask them to turn on the flashing lights, but I was too shy. *It's not really that important. It's not like I'm dying or something,* I told myself. When they opened the doors again, a blast of cold air shot in. I remember the small brown square tiles, like in a restaurant's kitchen, on the ramp leading into the hospital, and the sliding glass doors that opened silently before us under a sign that said, "South Hospital." I saw the reception desk because it was under a spotlight, but most of the rest of the hospital was dark. We went straight to the elevators. The elevators were *fast.* When the doors opened to the fourteenth floor, a small, long-faced man in a white coat and a bow tie stood waiting. The next thing I remember was waking up in a dark room that had three other kids in it, each separated by a curtain.

I was in the first bed to the right of the door, and in front of me, looking back, was another girl. She looked to be about my age, maybe a little older. I couldn't tell because it was kind of dark. I could tell, though, that she didn't have any hair, and she wore a black baseball cap. She smiled at us and said, "Hi, I'm Rachel." We all just looked at her, but she kept smiling. "Don't worry. They're the best up here. They'll figure it out in no time. It seems horrible right now, but everything will work out. Trust me."

I didn't say anything. I was too tired. Before I dropped off, I saw the thin man with the bow tie wearing the very short white coat enter the room, hands in the coat pockets.

"I'm Dr. Wolff."

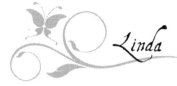

Linda

When we got to OHSU, I thought, Oh my God, this is big-time. *I was only thirty-two then, but I don't think* anyone *is mature enough to really process what's going on when you're dealing with news like this. When we got there I thought I was in hell. The ward looked dirty, dingy, and depressing. The walls were brown. There were spare beds and wheelchairs and equipment overflowing into the hallway. Everything looked like a mess. It felt like a time warp because so much of the design looked like it jumped out from the 1940s. Oh, I was in hell.*

I just remembered thinking that people sent their kids to Doernbecher because something was seriously, seriously wrong. I thought Dr. Wolff was—everything was just, like, so alien. This guy I didn't even know was way too brilliant for me to even talk to. He assigned me homework. I was learning about all this stuff I didn't know—stuff I didn't ever want to know—and I had to read these texts and articles again and again and again before I could understand what in God's name he was talking about and what the right decisions could be. The worst part of this whole process was everything that led up to the confirmed diagnosis because it was just all so uncertain. The anticipation of test results can be cruel.

It took a few days to realize how good Doernbecher was. The fear factor was so strong, and the shock factor of everything we were enduring was just too much for us to really appreciate everything around us. When Wolff started giving us statistics and information about the disease, we started to feel better. It wasn't so bad once we had a name for it. Once we knew what to do about it.

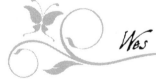

Wes

I was stunned by the antiquity of the hospital. Given the gravity of the work that the staff on this floor did, the facilities with which they did it just stunned me. There were rooms with four beds, rooms with two beds, and I think a total of two private rooms on the whole floor.

But Dr. Wolff was man with an aura of complete competence. At one point we finally just said to him, "What is going on?" He laid his suspicions and predictions all out for us that night—guesses that turned out to be the exact truth: "I think it's this type of disease, that is highly curable—odds about 95 percent in her favor." That put me 100 percent at ease right then and there. Yeah, there were some hoops we had to jump through, and they weren't going to be that pleasant, but she was going to be just fine. That was a huge relief to me. Linda, however, didn't take it so well so quickly. She worried a lot.

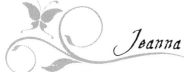

Jeanna

In the middle of that first night, we all get shuffled into this side, not-quite-a-conference room. There weren't enough chairs for everyone. Dr. Wolff stood up and offered his chair to me. I should have turned it down. He should have been able to sit. But I took it, and he started off with his ranked guesses. "My first guess is Wilms Tumor," and he talked about it with us.

My first impression of Dr. Wolff was that he was very smart. Very nerd-like doctor-ish. I absolutely knew that he knew what he was doing and that I could trust him absolutely. I mean, he came to us in the middle of the night! I was glad we were in a place where they didn't just sedate her and wait till morning.

Travis

I was only six, and I remember not knowing what was going on. Mom sent me over to Grandma's house to stay the night. Jeanna was acting weird. She seemed a little frantic. Worried about something. In the end, I was pretty jealous of Lindsey when I found out she got to ride in an ambulance.

Over the next several months we would always go see this guy, Dr. Wolff, all the time. I'd just learned the word "yuppie," but I didn't know what it meant, and so I walked in the door and said "Hello, Yuppie Wolff!" one day. Mom got pretty pissed. Dr. Wolff seemed to think it was funny. Sometimes the kids could really get him laughing and you could hear it echo down the halls.

Holly

I was watching TV with my brother Devin. My mom answered the phone and called me into the kitchen because it was for me. I sat down in the tall chair by the phone and listened to Lindsey tell me what happened. Her stomach hurt, she had to go by ambulance to the hospital, they found a tumor, they don't know what it is. I got that hot, prickly feeling that I get in my scalp when I'm nervous and scared.

Ah, and then the moment we all recall, of Devin doing the only thing he knows how to do to make people feel better. Jokes. In his best "Ahnold" voice he recited a line from Kindergarten Cop: "It's not a toom-ah." And I got pissed and yelled at him, "It is a tumor!"

That weekend was a blur. I don't remember if I stopped bleeding, but I must have slept most of the time. I certainly don't remember peeing again. I don't remember being out of bed. I vaguely remember being in ultrasound at one point, marveling at how they could discern anything in those screens full of white and gray noise, and that I was actually looking at my own guts.

My next memories were on Monday. Surgery was scheduled for nine o'clock in the morning. Just before nine, we received word that I'd been bumped. I thought, *Well, this must not be all that bad since they're making me wait.* I was hungry. I had learned that the night before surgery, the nurse always comes in and wakes you up, asking if you want anything to eat, explaining that after the twelve-hour deadline you can't eat because of the anesthesia. I'd said no, so, of course, the next morning, all I had at my disposal were ice chips.

Finally, the man in the green jacket showed up with the gurney. The green jacket meant the guy was from transportation. They had a whole department in this place just for shuttling people around. I had to put one of those backless gowns on. I was told to remove my nail polish, my watch, and any jewelry. "Why?" I asked.

"Because it's weird down there in surgery."

I didn't know what that meant. Was it some kind of vortex? Was there some kind of magnetic field or something down there that would break my watch? Or suck it right off my wrist? And the nail polish. Why would I have to remove that? Turns out, the reason is not nearly that dramatic. They make you remove your belongings so they don't get *stolen*, and the nail polish so they can tell whether or not your fingers are turning blue. I love the idea that you have to take your watch off so would-be criminals in the OR won't steal it but that it's perfectly OK for you to be down there, dead asleep, with said criminals lurking about.

The guy who gave me the gown said I had to take off everything, but I thought, *Surely, I can keep my underwear. Right? That would be totally weird to not wear underwear.* I was embarrassed to ask someone whether I could keep my undies, so I just made the executive decision to keep them on. And my hospital socks. I climbed up on the gurney and away we went.

The last thing I remember before going under was a half dozen people gowned and masked from head to toe, bustling around me. Sticking those sticky things on my chest—just like on TV!—clamping the plastic thing on my fingertip—the monitor immediately started showing squiggling lines—and putting the mask on my face. I had a brief moment of total anxiety. *They're going to suffocate me!* I remembered a girl at school had her tonsils out a couple years ago, and she said the air in the mask smelled so bad she couldn't stand it and she started kicking and screaming. Could something really smell *that* bad?

"Just breathe normally," said a masked voice, softly. The man who spoke was holding the plastic air mask on my face. I relaxed and breathed. It smelled fine; actually, it smelled kind of sweet. Cherries? No, not quite. Strawberries? Maybe. But it also smelled like the baking aisle at the grocery store. I breathed and looked around as best I could. The room had a couple giant lights above the table I was laying on—like the ones at the dentist except *huge*. The walls were covered in pale green tiles, and there were stainless steel cabinets everywhere. I could see the tops of air tanks out of the corner of my eye, right near my head, and lots of plastic tubing. I couldn't see any of the tools they would use. I was afraid to see them, but I also wanted to know what everything looked like.

I didn't know exactly what they were going to do, except that it had to do with the giant thing under my ribs. *Were they going to use a saw? How big would the knife be? Maybe they scoop things out with a big spoon.*

Then the air began to change. It suddenly smelled...plastic. The masked voice spoke again but he sounded much further away and he echoed, "Just keep breathing. How about five good breaths, huh?" I counted as I inhaled each time, wondering how it would feel to fall asleep. Did it happen fast? Would it take twenty minutes? It always takes a long time for me to fall asleep at night. *One...two...three...four...hey, this isn't so bad. There's no way this will put me to slee...*

"Lindsey, can you hear me? Lindsey, I need you to open your eyes. Lindsey, can you hear me? I need you to look at me."

What had happened? I was so tired. *I've only been sleeping for a few seconds, why would they wake me?* I opened my eyes. There was a woman standing above me. Who was she? Where was I? Then it came back: *she's a nurse. I'm in the hospital.* But I wasn't in the operating room anymore. Why? They couldn't be done yet. I'd only slept a few seconds.

But she said, "You're out of surgery. You're in recovery now. You did great. Do you have any pain?"

I shook my head. *There's no way they're done already. That only took, like, five seconds. Oh, who cares. I just want to sleep some more.*

"OK, then. You can go back to sleep now."

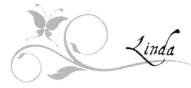

When your kid comes out of surgery, you get so caught up in emotions. My homework readings all said that kids mostly recover very well from things like surgery—better than a lot of adults do. But all that flies right out the window when you see your kid come out of surgery. It was hard. I don't do well when I'm in a dismal environment, so even though we had great care, I wasn't coping. The thought of someone cutting on my kid really messed me up.

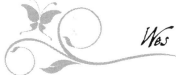

It's hard to look at somebody that close to you going through this kind of pain. At this time I personally had never had a surgery, so Lindsey was facing things that I had no idea about. I thought, How incredibly brave she is to say, "Let's go. Let's get this done." *Because I'd chickened out on a back surgery years before, thinking,* No way I'm going to let them put me under.

I opened my eyes. In front of me was a TV mounted on the wall near the ceiling. I was in one of those regular hospital beds again, in a two-person room. There were people next to me. Mom and Dad. I was near a window and felt very glad to have left the dark, four-person room behind (I never saw the girl in the black hat again). My window and the counter below it were covered in flowers, balloons, presents, cards, everything. It looked like my birthday and Christmas had thrown up all over.

Mom spoke up. "A lot of people have come to see you. They brought you all this stuff." I couldn't believe what I was seeing. It was way bigger than Christmas! Who knew that when you went to the hospital people give you presents?

Dad asked, "Hey, Boo, did you feel sick or anything when you woke up? From the anesthesia?" I shook my head. No, it was like waking up at home. They had told me I might feel nauseous or have a sore throat when I woke up. I didn't have any of those problems.

Then, without warning, I slept.

It appears that some critical things happened during a time period that is now only a black pall to me. Most of that weekend prior to surgery is a void. I believe that I have since blocked certain events from my own memory as a coping mechanism. I don't even remember if my kidney continued to bleed or if they managed to stop it somehow. From that vague trip to ultrasound, I sort of recall seeing in the monitor a fragment of tumor hanging out in the renal vein, flapping with every beat of my heart, threatening to detach and metastasize in some ungodly place. I have no memory of my allergic reaction to morphine—thus the reason for the Demerol—nor can I remember being informed by Dr. Wolff that I had Stage IV Wilms Tumor, a kidney cancer with very good cure rates, or that they considered my case to be an emergency and we could not afford to wait for a full recovery from the surgery before beginning treatment. Dad insists that I was lucid, that I acknowledged the gravity of the situation and commanded that we "get this thing outta me." They claim that I said we needed to fight this, and that I participated in these conversations in every way.

I have no memory of any of these things.

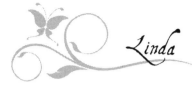

People don't know what to say when they figure out that you have cancer. It's kind of odd. All these different types of personalities come into play. Some people don't say anything. Some people say too much. Some people cry. Some people want to tell you their life story because they had a friend with cancer. And they don't realize that no two cancers are the same.

A lot of times, people judged us based on what our kid had. They'd shake their heads slowly and say, "Oh, you're so lucky you have that instead of what we have." And, yeah, we were lucky to have such a common, curable cancer, but that didn't make what we were experiencing any better. I didn't like the whole guilt thing, so we didn't get involved in a lot of organizations. Some people like Candlelighters, for instance, and it works really well for them because of the support network, but I just personally couldn't handle all the boohooing.

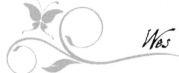

At one point, Lindsey asked Dr. Wolff, "What is this?" He looked at Linda and me questioningly. Linda said, "Be frank." So he told her it was a cancer, and some details of what they were planning to do for treatment. To my surprise, she said, "Let's go. Let's get this done. Get this out of me."

I awoke again. It was daylight. Was it still the same day? Was it tomorrow? How come I wasn't hungry? That couldn't be right. *Maybe I should make myself eat something.* I looked to my right and saw an IV pole there. I remembered an article I'd read at Sharon's house last summer: a boy had gotten suddenly very sick and had to go to the hospital. They said he had some kind of disease, and he had to have a big surgery, too. Afterward, the nurse told him they were going to feed him through a tube. Were they feeding me through my IV? What would they feed me? Could you puree burritos and put them in a tube? After reading that horrifying article, I'd thought, *Wow. I'm glad nothing like that could ever happen to me.*

I wished I could remember what disease he had. Maybe I had the same one.

Then I wondered, *What* did *happen to me?* They had never told me. Or maybe they did and I forgot. Or maybe they told Mom and Dad when I was sleeping. Maybe they didn't *want* me to know. Obviously this was a big deal: I was in a special hospital, I had this new doctor with a bow tie, and I'd just been cut open. *Cut open.* I lifted the blankets and pulled up the lovely magenta gown I was wearing. On my stomach, just above my belly button, was a line, a thin red line, stretching from side to side. *They almost cut me in half.* And stuck across it were little strips of tape! They cut me in half, and then they *taped* me back together! They could *do* that? I thought they stapled you or sewed you–like on the Frankenstein monster. Instantly I felt relieved that there were no staples involved, but I'd have to be careful about that tape. It might not stay stuck on very well, and then everything could fall out. God knows I'd had my problems with Scotch tape in the past.

OK, so I wasn't hungry, I didn't hurt, and…I hadn't peed in a long time. I looked up at the IV. They were pumping some pretty fat bags of water through me. *Why wasn't I peeing?* I felt my hips. My underwear was gone. *Oh my God. Where did it go? Did they undress me while I was asleep? Why? Can they legally* do *that?* Then I saw it: a clear plastic tube poking out under the blankets that went over the side of the bed. I could see it had pale yellow liquid in it. I shifted in the bed and two things happened simultaneously. I felt something odd between my legs and thought, *That must be the tube.* The tube actually was stuck into my bladder. Briefly, I thought, *How do they do that?*

Then the pain flared up, interrupting my thoughts. But "flare" doesn't even begin to describe it. I had tried to flex abdominal muscles that had just been severed. They screamed at me in wrenching pain. My breath caught and I uttered a small sound, which also caused pain in my throat. My hand went to my face and felt another tube. *There was a tube in my nose.* I felt for it on the bed. It went down to a plastic container on the IV pole, and little spongy bits of green and yellow flowed through it. *It's sucking stuff out of me.* The little pump made a soft droning noise.

I tried to process all this new information. To my left, Mom was sleeping. Near her were stacks of papers and books. *What time is it? What day is it?* On the other side of the curtain, I heard someone rustling around. So I had a neighbor. I could see the glow from the hallway and hear the general bustle of people and phones. Was it early? I looked outside. Typical Portland overcast day. No help there.

I waited, my stomach still pretty painful. Tears sat in the corners of my eyes, waiting. Then I heard someone enter the room. A few someones. Three white-coats entered my side of the room. One was my doctor with the bow tie, Dr. Wolff. A very lean man, he was maybe in his early fifties and had a long face in which his brown eyes exuded extreme intelligence and at the same time seemed very weary. His eyebrows were monstrous. I mean *huge.* Think Groucho Marx, but bushier. Dr. Wolff had a terse but not unpleasant personality. He walked around with his hands in his coat pocket, thumbs sticking out. The man next to him was tall and slightly husky with graying hair and eyeglasses. He seemed to grin perpetually. He was very amiable, and his coat was very long. There was a woman, too. She had short blond hair and thick gold earrings pierced high up on the ridges of her ears. The earrings were distracting; I found myself staring helplessly at them when she talked, wondering if they pierced through the hard part of her ear or just clipped around it. She had a long stark white coat and accompanying humorless, caustic personality.

How come Wolff wore this tiny coat that showed off his hips and these other guys had these big long coats? "Morning," said Dr. Wolff. He indicated the tall man. "This is Dr. Norman, and this is Dr. Stein," he finished, gesturing to the woman. They were colleagues. So, in a way, they were all my doctors. Three docs. What was going on?

They asked if I felt sick or had any pain. I nodded, still feeling the burn from that earlier movement. They wanted to know from one to ten, ten being the worst, what my pain was. "Six," I whispered.

"Mmhmm. Mmhmm." Dr. Wolff nodded perfunctorily. "OK, we can take care of that." Then they all wanted to see the line. I lifted my gown, careful to keep all of my privates covered. They said it looked good. I asked what the tube in my nose was for. Dr. Wolff answered, "It's pulling any acid and lining that might detach from your stomach out of you." He explained that abdominal surgery throws everything out of whack, and it takes awhile for the body to get everything right again. That vacuum tube kept me from feeling too sick by sucking the bad stuff out. I looked at the tube. So the green bits were *stomach lining*. I couldn't decide if that was neat or gross.

"How about you to get up and take a walk today. Can you do that?" He looked at me expectantly with those eyebrows pointed skyward, revealing lines on his forehead as they went. I shrugged. He pointed toward the hall as he turned to walk out. "I'll go tell the nurse. We'll be back later."

So I had to get up today. I remembered how shifting in bed hurt so badly and wondered if getting up would feel the same.

Oh, yes.

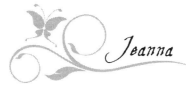

Jeanna

I remember sitting by Lindsey one day, and she was just feeling kind of blue. She had tubes down her throat and couldn't really talk. I asked her, "You know you're going to be all right, don't you?" She wrote on a piece of paper, "Yes. After kimo." First I thought of Kemosabe and The Lone Ranger, wondering what she meant. Then I thought, Oh, gosh. Kids have to deal with chemo and they don't even know how to spell the word.

I spent nights in the hospital, never leaving her alone, because that was the one piece of advice that had been given to me by a friend. Never leave them alone.

In a word, getting up was horrible. I sincerely doubt there exists worse pain. Breech childbirth can't be this bad. The nurse came in and announced that we were going to stand up, turn around, and sit in the chair next to the bed so she could put a foam egg crate pad under the sheets. That didn't seem like it should be such a big deal. I could do that. But from the moment she, Mom and Jeanna began to help me pull myself out of bed the pain hit like a tsunami. All other thoughts and feelings fled my mind. Only pain existed and only pain mattered. I felt like I couldn't breathe. I tried to scream, but doing so was even more painful. This was the hardest lesson in gross anatomy—you need your abs to scream.

Who ever knew the simple movement that we normally take for granted—standing, turning, and sitting again—would require three assistants and take an eternity? The whole thing probably took between three and five minutes at the most, but for me, each second was a lifetime. My stomach felt as if an unseen hand was using a red-hot iron poker to continually slice me. My throat stung from screaming and that awful tube. I shudder to think of what the other children on the floor thought when they heard me.

Suddenly, a blessed reprieve: I was in the chair, sweating and completely out of breath. The pain that had been like a white hot blast furnace had burned down to pulsing embers and finally cooled to a mere echo—so long as I didn't move so much as an eyelash, not to mention shift my weight from one cheek to another. Rigidly, I watched one of the nurses make the bed, dreading my next movement, thinking that I'd never seen a bed made so quickly. My back started to hurt from tension.

Suddenly, anger flared up within me, as hotly as my body had just felt it was burning moments before. Why didn't they have this bed ready for me when I came back from surgery? How could they be so inept? And then to make me suffer for it!

Someone–I don't remember if it was the nurse or mom or Jeanna–took hold of my hands to brace my weight to stand. I started to cry. It hurt, and I cried harder from the pain. My anger and hatred immediately replaced by profound terror, I pleaded, "Don't make me do it. I can't do it." I sobbed, feeling the hot tears roll down my cheeks. "Please don't. Please, it's the worst pain. I can't stand it."

"One to ten where is your pain?"

I paused momentarily. "Twelve."

"Are you sure? It's the worst pain of your life?"

What, were they thick? Would this lady like me to cut *her* in half and then make her walk around? I looked at her and nodded.

"We have to get you back in bed," she said. "You can sit here a little longer if you like, but eventually you need to go back."

I was cold. I wanted to be in my blankets. How long could I endure cold toes just to stay in the chair? Then another thought occurred: *Is this what torture feels like?* It must be. In the movies you always saw people begging for it to stop. I'd tell them anything they wanted to hear if they would make it stop.

"Come on, let's get you in bed. You can do it; we'll go real slow. We'll put you back in the blankets and you can sleep. How's that sound?" Good old Mom trying to encourage me. She couldn't possibly understand.

Actually, she could. Unbeknownst to me, Mom had her gall bladder removed when I was a wee one. Back then, they did a huge open abdominal surgery similar to what had just been done to me. She knew what it felt like all right.

"Yeah," the nurse added. "We'll go see about getting you something more to control your pain." That sounded like a gimmick to me, but I could see no alternative. And so we started back. The twenty inches spanning the distance between the bed and me stretched out as long and as arduous as the Tour de France. With every movement I felt I was being disemboweled. Finally, I lowered myself into the bed, exhausted. It *was* more comfortable with the egg crate.

"Next time, let's get you a folded blanket or a pillow or something to use as a support against your tum-tum, OK?" Mom suggested, tucking me in.

Brilliant. Why didn't you people think of that before we started this?

Mom spoke up again. "Booie, every time you do this, it'll get easier and easier. Moving helps you heal faster."

What was that supposed to mean, "every time"? How often did they think I was gonna do this? The nurse came back in and injected something into the IV.

Night-night.

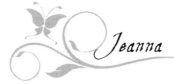

Jeanna

I don't know how, but the word got out to the community because when I went to work on Monday, I said something about Lindsey being in the hospital and needing surgery, and the hygienist said, "Oh, my neighbor said there was a girl who came to the hospital who thought she started her period but it was a tumor." How do people know this stuff?

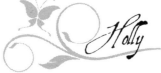

Holly

I remember going with my mom to see Lindsey for the first time on 14A. Chatting, acting like sixth graders. Then, when we left, my mom sat me down in the lobby on the first floor to talk, and I knew exactly what she was going to say, even though deep inside I didn't want her to say it.

"Holly, Lindsey has cancer."

I ran into the bathroom and sat in the stall and sobbed. I cried because I was scared for her, what she was going to go through. I was a little scared she would die, that I would lose my best friend, but I also knew that wasn't true. My brain has a way of getting news and fast-forwarding that news months or years ahead. I didn't just see the immediate shock; I saw the hospital stays, chemo, sickness, weakness, how people would treat her.

Life in the hospital is a curious routine. You get used to daily rhythms quickly: morning rounds, vitals every four hours, breakfast, housekeeping, school, lunch and dinner trays, evening rounds, and the arrival and departure of the nursing staff. The nurses are profound. Our very first nurse was named Bancy, and she had the most exotic accent I'd ever heard–South African, maybe–it perfectly accessorized her enormous radiant smile and twinkling eyes. Mom was never quite able to say her name properly. It always came out "Bouncy." The second was Denise. Denise looked a lot like Jeanna, and she was very devoted my care, very thorough. She always came running quickly when I called for her, and she went about her business—even the most unenjoyable jobs, like emptying the urine bag—with joy and satisfaction. She made me feel more comfortable than anyone else and was assigned to me every evening. I started to request her to be sure I didn't get stuck with some stranger.

"How about that Dr. Wolff, huh?" she asked me one night, smiling, as she injected my meds. "What a guy. Those bow ties, aren't they great?" I had never thought about Dr. Wolff as being "what a guy," but now I did. I smiled. Those bow ties *were* great.

Every morning, a short, old Asian woman came in to change the linens. It was just another opportunity to get me out of bed. Here was a woman who loved her job, really. She would knock quietly on the door and shuffle in, sheets folded neatly over one arm, singing, "Good moorning, Lin-say!" Those were the only words she ever said to me. We'd get me out of bed, and she would take over with the utmost efficiency, folding the sheets with perfect "hospital corners"; and then, before I knew it, I would be back in bed, tucked in, and she would shuffle out, smiling all the while and not to be seen until the next morning.

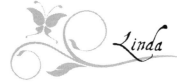

Linda

Everyone hears the word cancer *and they immediately unravel. It still does that to me until I stop and think about it. In a lot of situations, cancer doesn't mean a death sentence. When we were first diagnosed, and they said the word* cancer, *I thought,* Oh my god, cancer. That only happens to older people. And they die. *I had no education in it, and I had no reason to think otherwise.*

After we started going through the process, I started to learn that death wasn't automatic. As the tests and scans came back, there were a lot of things to be positive about, and I began to realize Lindsey could go on to live a normal life.

I thought Tylenol was completely stupid. I couldn't believe they expected me to take Tylenol to control my pain two days out of surgery. Here I was, hooked to every tube and machine out there, and they were giving me *Tylenol?* Doctors must get money or something to endorse Tylenol because it does precisely jack for post-surgery pain. If you have a *headache,* take Tylenol. If you've just been sliced 'n' diced, you need something more powerful. Excedrin. No, seriously. So they gave me this machine that would provide almost an endless stream Demerol. I could self-administer every ten minutes if I needed. A real junkie's dream. The problem with Demerol is that it does little more than Tylenol to control major pain. If anything, I felt worse. Not only could I still feel everything, it made me restless and spacey. I couldn't sleep when I wanted and couldn't stay awake when I had to. Eventually, they gave me thick red capsules that seemed to soften both the pain and the world around me a bit.

People came to visit: teachers, classmates, friends, relatives. Some visits were good. Others, not so much. One night, some classmates and my math teacher, Sister Alice, came up. Mom woke me, and I saw them standing at the foot of the bed, looking at me, trying to smile at me but looking more like deer in the headlights, grimacing in fear. There was enough time to see them and process who they were before the pain hit. The meds had worn off. I started to scream and cry. The girls' eyes suddenly became as wide as saucers; they gasped as they were ushered quickly into the hallway. Someone ran for the nurse, who came rushing in with one of those red pills. I managed to swallow it, and it took about ten minutes to take hold. Finally, Mom went to find my guests, and they tentatively edged their way back in, looking at me as if I had just brandished a large weapon at them.

I couldn't keep track of time very well. Though still not hungry, I kept thinking I should be eating, and asked for Jell-O. But no one else seemed to think that was right. The docs came and went twice a day—always in packs, except once Dr. Wolff appeared by himself in the doorway. He explained he had to dash off, but he wanted to let us know that the pathologist said it was "favorable histology." I had no idea what that meant, but Mom sighed audibly, saying, "Thank God," so I took it for a good thing.

I marked time by the appearances of my docs, but they weren't always punctual. The students would come in the early morning, nudge you awake, and ask how you'd been sleeping. They were always asking about "bowel movements" and "flatulence." If you said yes when they asked you if you'd experienced either in the last twenty-four hours, they'd look at each other almost triumphantly and be very excited. As for my trio of oncologists, sometimes they accompanied the students, sometimes not. I started to really like Dr. Norman and Dr. Wolff a lot. Dr. Wolff wore a different bow tie every day, and these were no clip on ties–he tied these himself, which I found very impressive. I had never seen any bow ties that didn't clip on. Dr. Norman had a tie with ice creams on it, which he'd bought at the original Ben & Jerry shop in New Jersey. We called it his "tasteful tie." Groan.

Mom was right. Over time, moving around became a little easier. I also figured out how to move without engaging my abs all the time. As for that tube in my throat, it became so uncomfortable that I took to writing instead of speaking whenever possible, and whispering when it wasn't. Everyone seemed to think I was just being silly, saying that I shouldn't feel the tube at all. But really, what did *they* know? It was installed in *me*.

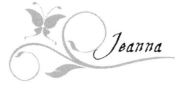

Jeanna

One day, post-surgery, it was just Lindsey and me in the room, and she wasn't feeling very good. Suddenly, she just burst out sobbing, saying, "I didn't want any of this to happen!" I held her and felt the hot tears roll down my cheek. I didn't dare sob, but I couldn't stop the tears. This was the lowest point of the whole thing.

A few days after surgery, after I'd only stood up a couple times, a nurse came in and put a big syringe full of yellow liquid in the IV drip. I watched, wondering if it was some kind of food. I hoped it was juice. It kind of looked like juice. Could you put juice in your veins? Maybe it was liquid food, like what the old people drink. Then again, it also looked like urine.

Several hours later, I figured out it most certainly was *not* food, as I violently pitched forward and vomited into a pink plastic tub, so eloquently dubbed an "emesis basin." The sudden forward movement caused an explosion of pain. This was as of yet not experienced. I was dealing with a whole new pain. Combined with the clenching of my stomach, I was in a right state. I moaned in pain, making a half-gargling, half-warbling sound because of the vomiting. This wasn't food. This was *chemotherapy*, a term with which I was not yet familiar. Having no suitable remedy for this side effect, they gave me two pills: Reglan and Benadryl. Trying to keep them down was a task in itself. Then, their effect took hold and I slept it off. So really, if I wasn't knocked out from the pain meds, I was knocked out from the Reglan and Benadryl.

I woke up one day and took stock of my situation. Here I was, barely able to move. I'd just been sliced and diced by a bunch of strangers. They were feeding me poison. I had a not one, but a *team* of doctors now, and this was obviously a very big deal. But why? What did I have? Suddenly, I wondered, *Am I going to die?* They had brought the priest in with the Eucharist to bless me and hear my confession before surgery. The Sacrament of the Anointing of the Sick. Once known as Extreme Unction, it was the blessing the Church gave you *right before you died.* Not to mention I felt like I might be dying, I was in so much pain. I knew I should ask Mom and Dad. But how? How do you ask your parents if you're dying? And what would they say if I was? What would I say? Would they lie to me? Everyone around me was clearly wigged out. I was afraid that if I asked someone, they would start crying. Then I would cry. And I was tired of crying. Then I'd be really scared. I decided the best plan would be to wait it out. If I was still here after Christmas, I'd be fine. I nodded to myself in agreement.

That's a good plan.

Later, the nurse again injected the chemo. I watched in antici-pation as the yellow liquid slowly crept toward my body through the clear plastic tube. Like clockwork, about six hours later, I heaved stomach acid into the plastic tub, which Dad and I named "the chunder chalice"—*chunder* from the Australian slang for "to barf" and *chalice* from my Catholic schooling meaning "vessel [of Christ's blood]." Except that chalices are generally gold or silver goblets, and this one was a pink plastic tub. Not exactly something in which one would celebrate the miracle of Transubstantiation.

And, like clockwork, they gave me another Reglan and Benadryl.

More time passed. They removed my urine catheter. It was the most peculiar feeling. It didn't really hurt. Not exactly. I was afraid when they told me what they were going to do, and I asked what it would feel like. You know, so I was braced for it. I didn't want anymore painful surprises. The nurse described it as a "sensation." I didn't know what that meant. She was right, though. It was a very peculiar feeling when the balloon passed from the bladder through the urethra and popped out. I didn't scream or cry, but I probably had crossed eyes.

After it was out, I felt like I had to pee every ten minutes. Dr. Wolff explained that because they'd been digging around in my abdominal cavity, poking, prodding, checking things out, my body had to readjust. So, what I was feeling was the "I gotta pee" nerves reacclimatizing. It turned out to be a good thing, too. They offered to put a commode in my room, but I refused, so I found myself getting up frequently and walking out to the only bathroom on the ward. I'm sure it sped the healing process.

After another while, one of the surgical residents came in and helped me roll onto my stomach. "All right. We are going to take out your epidural." Having no idea what an epidural was, I asked how much it would hurt.

"It should be painless."

They were very loose with the word "should." I didn't like it.

"We have to take some tape off, but you shouldn't feel the needle pull out at all." I did feel the sting of tape slowly being pulled away. Next thing I knew he was helping me roll onto my back again. He showed me a little needle. I couldn't believe that thing was in my spine.

"Let's have a look at that tube in your schnoz now, huh?" He inspected the little pump, still droning away, and the bits of green cruising through the tube. Finally, he said, "It'll be awhile yet until that one can come out." I explained it hurt to talk with that thing in there. "It shouldn't," he dismissed me. I stared at him. *Well lah-tee-dah, Dr. Smarty.*

One night, when Jeanna was taking a shift with me and after I'd had a sponge bath (it felt incredible—the hot washcloth scrubbing against tired skin. I never knew a bath could feel so heavenly), Mom came in with a shopping bag. "Booie! Look what I got you!" She set the bag down and started to pull stuff out of it. "Some "nightgowns..." One was white with blue polka dots—it almost looked like the hospital gowns—one was lavender with flowers, and another was bright yellow with a big Tweety Bird face on the front. She continued, "I got you some scrunchies for your hair…" She pulled out a pack of three, red, white, and blue. "…and some nail polish!" She revealed a bag of cotton balls, acetone, and a few shades of nail polish. "I thought that since you're all squeaky clean we'll have some beauty time. Now, which nightgown do you want?"

"They just gave me a new gown. I don't want to stand up again," I said firmly. I had been contemplating whether or not I'd feel a difference in pain levels now that they'd taken that thing out of my back. So far so good, but I wasn't about to take any chances.

"OK, we'll save it for the next time you get up," she said, stuffing them back into the bag. "Here," she handed me the nail polish, "pick a color. How about I brush your hair out all nice and Jeanna can paint your toes?" I raised the head of my bed as far as it would go, and Jeanna pulled my treaded socks off and took the red polish I'd chosen. She pushed cotton balls between my toes and started to paint. She managed to get about half on the nails and half on my cuticles, laughing, "I'm not very good at painting toes!" Mom had taken the hairbrush and was brushing out my tangles. It felt good for the little wire bristles to scratch against my scalp. When she was done brushing, she pulled my hair back in a high pony and wrapped it with the white scrunchie. Between the two of them, Mom and Jeanna managed to clean most of the wayward polish from my cuticles. I'll admit, I was the cutest post-nephrectomy, pre-alopecia chemo patient *ever*.

More time passed. I began to walk the hallways on the ward. Making a full loop was the goal. The first time, Jeanna and Mom were my assistants. We slowly shuffled out the door, Jeanna helping me stand, support blanket thrust firmly against my stomach, which I feared would rip open if I so much as stumbled or veered off balance. Mom minded the IV pole that Jeanna had dubbed "Stand-ley, our Pole-ish friend," and hanging from Stand-ley's "head" on a pink ribbon was a sign written in pink cursive that said, "Lindsey's Health Juice" courtesy of my best friend Holly.

In front of the nurse's desk was the whiteboard listing every patient on the ward and his or her doctors. Jeanna stopped and said, "Let's see if we can find your name, Boo."

We stopped to look.

Mom didn't notice.

Presently, I felt my IV and the suction tube start pulling. Hard. I inhaled brusquely as I shuffled forward to relieve the tension. The sudden movement brought fresh, hot tears to my eyes and a hard, burning feeling at the back of my throat. My abs groaned in pain. I groaned in pain. Mom stopped short when she heard me.

"Why did you keep going?" I shrieked, eyes brimming.

She looked back at me, shocked. "I didn't know you stopped!" She was clearly distressed. There wasn't any time to go on. I suddenly had an overwhelming urge to vomit again, with no chunder chalice in sight. I couldn't stand the idea of just throwing up on the floor in front of everyone.

Mom saw instantly. "You think you're gonna throw?" she asked. I nodded. The thought of throwing up again made the tears worse. My eyes were swimming. The ward was a blur.

"I think it's your stomach pump," Jeanna said. We rushed, as quickly and gracefully as sea turtles waddling in the sand, back to the room to plug in the pump. Mom snapped my end of the hose back into the machine. It chugged to life, and I could see more green matter than ever flying through the tube. Immediately, I could feel the nauseous pressure lifting. I realized that I wasn't just aiming to walk the loop; I now had a time trial against my stomach pump.

Finally, the day came when I was able to eat. Problem was, I didn't want to. The food would come, bringing with it a heavy, pungent, unpleasant aroma. One time a strange-looking hot dog showed up. It looked sweaty. The bun looked like plastic. I took one look and thought, *Right. I don't think so.* My grammie–mom's mom–was there, and she chortled, "Oh, but Lindsey! It comes with *fries!*" Actually, it was the fries that reeked the worst. Grammie loves her french fries though. As long as I could remember, whenever we went out to eat, she would always say, "Lindsey, get something with fries for your old Grammie." I was happy to oblige.

This time however, fries or not, lunch was a no-go. "You can have them," I said to her.

Linda

I actually wanted one of the other doctors on the oncology team instead of Dr. Wolff. I wanted Dr. Norman. That didn't have anything to do with good decision making; he just looked more warm and cuddly. More of a grandfatherly figure. In actuality, Dr. Wolff was just a godsend. I can't imagine having any other oncologist in his place.

Dr. Wolff wasn't all warm and cuddly. That made this transition hard. Because that's what you want when you're going through cancer: someone who'll tuck you in and say, "Everything will be OK." But once we started breaking through the shell with him, he became a different person. When he warmed up to you, things looked better. I asked him once about some worrisome statistics that I'd come across in my "homework," and he said, "Yeah, I wouldn't put as much credence into that data. The best thing is to talk to some of our other patients who have done well with this. Remember that statistics are just generalizations. Every person's experience is different."

About day seven after surgery, a pack of docs entered. One of them was the same guy who had removed my epidural.

"Time for your schnoz tube to go!" he announced. This was my last tube (I didn't think the IV really counted as a "tube"). The others watched while he undid the tape.

"OK, I'm going to count to three; then I want you to totally relax your throat and hold your breath. It'll make this a lot easier." He paused. "Oh, and you'll probably want to blow your nose after." On three, I held my breath and braced myself. He pulled. And pulled. And pulled. I stared down, crossing my eyes at the thing coming out my nose. I could feel it moving inside. Hand over hand, he pulled. Finally, I felt it give and it was out completely. Then, my head felt very full. Dad handed over a tissue. I blew and took it away from my face. It was still connected to my face by a thick rope of clear, shiny mucous. I began to spin the tissue, winding the snot around and around.

Everyone in the room continued to observe intently, comically. Still it kept winding.

Then it snapped free. My head felt *clean* on the inside—so clean it stung to take a breath. I spoke. No more pain. I sighed relief. Inwardly, I thought smugly about how I was right after all about that stupid tube. I handed the tissue to a gloved nurse.

I felt good for the first time in a week.

Now, free of all tubes except the IV, I played a game of pool with my cousins one night. I found that so long as I moved slowly and very deliberately, I could make it work. It was a shot in the arm–a good one for once–to play with my cousins. Mom followed me around and watched like a hawk to make sure I didn't rip out the IV by accident. But it felt *normal* to be playing such a *normal* game with my *normal* cousins. To call it a relief would be an understatement.

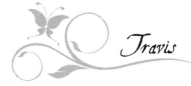

Travis

I got scared a little from what was going on, but not scared for Lindsey so much. I was scared that something might happen to me, somehow. One day, Mom asked me if I understood what was happening, and if I was afraid of anything. I said, "I'm afraid I might lose my play buddy."

Jeanna

Linda told me that in the car on the way home from the hospital one day, Travis turned to her and said, "Lindsey, are you going to die?"

Day nine. I was going home! All my tubes and the IV were gone. I'd made five laps around the ward that morning. I was still afraid to walk without someone next to me or without using my blanket brace, so they were letting me take it home with me.

It took the big red Radio Flyer several trips to cram all my stuff into the car. I was wearing new clothes. Mom had bought stretch pants for me with soft elastic waists so that I didn't hurt my incision, like I was afraid I would on a regular old pair of jeans.

Dad blocked the biting November wind as I carefully, slowly hoisted myself from the wheelchair to the front seat of the car. *Nice,* I thought, *I get the front seat!* Then we hit a snag: the seatbelt. It hit the critical area.

"I don't want to wear it. It'll hurt me," I said.

"You're wearing it," Dad mandated, wagging his finger at me. "We're not coming back here for more if we get in an accident." In the end, we shielded my front with the trusty support blanket and buckled up. When I walked into my room that night, the ceiling was full of dozens of balloons, courtesy of my grammie.

Linda

    I was so thankful for our friend Sharon's husband, Dr. Dogan, who was an oncologist for adults at Tuality Hospital. He told me, "Read everything you can get your hands on. Absolutely everything." Reading really gave me power and security. I read about things I'd never heard of. I didn't want to, but I did it and it was the right thing to do. I came to the conclusion that you can either break down and not be good for anybody, or you can buck up and be strong and get stuff done.

    I was not only trying to make decisions for Lindsey and my husband and son, but I was also trying to console family members, friends, and even the staff at Lindsey's school. People would get so worked up over the most inaccurate information. Rumors flew. I finally had to stand back and say, "Look, you don't know what you're talking about, and you can get the information from me and we can do the right thing, or you can stay away while we deal with this."

Wes

    Linda has this ability to do absolutely anything that has to be done as soon as she realizes that she has to do it. Underneath her city-girl exterior, she has grit equal to that of any pioneer.

    Until this horror, there had only been one major hospital situation when Lindsey was about two years old when we thought she'd swallowed a whole bottle of aspirin. We took her to the doctor and they were trying to force ipecac or something down her throat to make her throw up. It wasn't working very well, and we had to help hold her down. Linda was crying and inconsolable. At one point I finally said to her, "Enough. If you can't control yourself, you need to leave the room. This is hard enough as it is." To my utter amazement she instantly shut it off and did what had to be done. Lindsey could not have had a more perfect mother to help her through cancer.

I enjoyed a little time off after I came home from Doernbecher. I recovered my sense of humor as I healed, and began to feel somewhat normal again. But we weren't out of the woods yet. We now had to finish the treatments, which meant we would be at the Oregon Health and Science University clinics a lot from here on out.

It felt like we'd been walking forever, winding in endless fluorescent circles. This place was a big ant farm. My stomach was reeling from the odor on the first floor from the coffee bar. That smell permeated every hallway and every room, clinging to carpet fibers, the walls, even people's clothes. We passed a number of different offices: Women's Health/Obstetrics, down the hall; Otolaryngology/Ear, Nose and Throat around the corner; Nephrology...I stared at the patterns of linoleum on the floor. Finally, we found the right clinic: Pediatric Hematology/Oncology. The waiting room was dark and crammed full of people. There was no place to sit. When we were called back, I met some new nurses: Patsy and Kaylee, who would become central figures in my treatment. I became familiar with what would soon be automatic routine: check-in, remove shoes, weight check, height check, BP check, and temperature. The thermometers were thin plastic strips, with little capsules on one end that read the temperature. I couldn't avoid playing with the capsules with my tongue—once I broke one with my teeth and it spilled foul-tasting liquid onto my tongue. Then we went to a room and waited for Dr. Wolff. Sometimes I could hear other kids screaming through the walls, and I wondered if whatever it was that was being done to them would be done to me next.

Dr. Wolff appeared. That man had a knack for appearing. I never seemed to see him arrive; he always managed to silently arrive, and I thought, *How did you get here?* That day, thick binder in hand, he went over my treatment protocol in detail. We agreed to be part of the National Wilms Tumor Study that was comparing the effectiveness of two different treatments: one long and one short. My treatment plan would have a few phases, which we had already started in the hospital. The first phase would consist of twelve weeks of Vincristine, given every Monday intravenously, and radiation therapy to my chest and abdomen until the tumors in my lungs were gone and they felt they'd hit the "tumor bed" hard enough (I pictured something like a giant lima bean wearing a fuzzy nightcap, sleeping on a four-poster bed with pink satin blankets).

The drugs were funny. They had two names. One was given by the pharmaceutical company, and one was its scientific name. Dr. Wolff generally used the scientific name. After the first twelve weeks, they would begin alternating between cycles of Adriamycin (scientific name doxorubicin) and actinomycin D (scientific name Dactinomycin) until we reached the six-month mark. Then, the study's central computer would flip a coin of sorts to decide whether I was home free or whether I would continue to the fifteenth-month mark.

Dr. Wolff encouraged me to have all this done as an outpatient, so I could go home to my own bed and be as normal as possible. He encouraged me to spend time with my pets and go to school, saying that they would help normalize things.

The chemo experience didn't end with the drugs and the constant throwing up, as most of the public is familiar with. I wouldn't see the dentist again until treatment was over, and while on treatment I wasn't supposed to use a regular toothbrush. They informed us that I could easily cause my gums to bleed, and if the platelet counts were low enough I might not stop. Instead, they gave me these things that looked like little pink suckers. They were sponges on a stick that tasted vaguely like fluoride. Dr. Wolff informed us that I might also get nosebleeds, and if I did I wasn't supposed to tip my head back when I plugged my nose. Leg cramps were another possibility. He also said that not every patient loses his or her hair. "Did ya hear that, Booie? You might not lose your hair!" Mom exclaimed. She patted my hand reassuringly. I thought, *That would be great!* But I had a feeling that Dr. Wolff expected my hair to go, and so it probably would.

After we'd discussed all the logistics, it was time for Vincristine. Patsy came in with a metal tray lined with what looked like a really thick paper towel. On the paper towel was the rubber tourniquet, alcohol swabs, a few glass vials with rubber tops of different colors, a large syringe full of dark yellow liquid, a syringe with clear liquid, a cotton ball, and a little plastic container inside which something was coiled. She started getting everything ready to go. The thing inside the plastic container was the needle. It was very thin, but also long, and on either side of the needle were little green plastic "wings", and so it was referred to as a butterfly needle. I thought it looked more like a big mosquito. Connected to the needle was a long thin tube with a socket on the end to which they would screw the syringes. *How appropriate,* I thought, *that this thing coils up like a snake.* The smell of alcohol permeated the air, and she came at my arm.

Three nurses, two hotpacks, and several failed butterflies later, Dr. Wolff came in to do the job. He was able to find a vein with less difficulty than the others, but it was no small task. My face was red and tear-streaked by the time he got a blood return in the butterfly, at which point I was finally able to visibly relax. He drew enough blood to fill the glass vials on the tray. Then, in went the clear syringe. He pushed half of its contents through the butterfly. I felt a mild salty taste in my mouth. In went the yellow syringe. I stared at where the butterfly needle tucked under my skin while he slowly injected it, then the first syringe went back in and flushed the remaining yellow liquid through the tube. He pressed the cotton ball over the top while he pulled the butterfly out and firmly affixed the Barbie Band-Aid.

Simple as that.

It felt weird that it was that simple to get chemo. Wolff sent us home with an appointment for next Monday and scripts for Reglan, Benadryl, and a new drug called sulfamethoxazole (commonly known as Septra or sulfa), an antibiotic to help prevent infections. And so it went this way. Come in once for chemo, once for a blood count, and as often as the doctors in the radiation department mandated, every week.

Vincristine was funny. Over time, I noticed that the upper range of my voice almost totally disappeared. If I tried to yell at Travis or scream in pain, I was reduced to a silent hiss. It was scary having no voice. I could get tongue-twisted pretty easily, too. When Dr. Wolff would see me, he tested my tongue: "Say 'Methodists and Episcopalians.'" Sometimes I could do it just fine. Others, it would come out as "Methodith of Epis-Espisthcpalen." Then I would feel stupid for not being able to say it right. My tongue just felt like it was in the way all the time. Sometimes, I would have a hard time holding spoons, forks, or knives properly and would fist them like a child. Mom would get irritated and try to make me hold them correctly. Generally, they'd squirm out from between my fingers and clatter on the plate. It was the same with pencils and pens at school, and forget about scissors. Whenever this would happen, it always felt like the top two sections of my fingers just wanted to be straight all the time.

Radiation was a mixed bag of easy, comfortable, and embarrassing. It was quiet in the radiation department. It was dark. You can find quiet, dark places all over the world these days. They're called *spas*. But I wouldn't be getting massages or microdermabrasion here. The first time, they walked me into the treatment room, which was not unlike an OR. There was a table in the middle of the room, except instead of a giant light above me, there was what looked like an X-Ray machine. This was where the embarrassing part started.

They instructed me to remove my shirt and lie on the table. I looked at Mom and the doctor and a line of faces behind a window in the control room. *Seriously? I'm supposed to lay here all naked in front of you guys? In front of my* Mom? They waited expectantly. I sighed inwardly and pulled the shirt up over my head, revealing my tiny bra—barely more than a training bra. They helped me on the table and said that the bra had to go, too. As I reached behind to unclasp it, I ran a mantra through my head: *They're doctors. They do this all the time. It's OK. They're doctors. Yours are not the first boobs they've seen. The sooner you start, the sooner they'll be done. It's OK. They're doctors...*

I lay there on the table and became painfully aware of how cool the room was. I flushed as my nipples stood up. Nobody even batted an eye. The X-ray light turned on, casting its template over me. They drew a grid on my chest with a permanent marker, admonishing me not to so much as twitch while they did so. "We'll give you this pen," they said, "so you can retrace the lines as they fade. We need the grid to be exactly the same every time, so we don't hurt anything but the tumors." When they were done, someone took photos. I was horrified that pictures of my naked torso were going to be filed away somewhere. Probably where lots of people would see them.

The actual process of radiation therapy in my case was no big deal. They turned the light on, lined up the grid, and fired away. After the last nurse or doctor went behind the glass, they would once again admonish me to hold perfectly still, and the machine clicked on. It made a low buzzing sound for about thirty seconds or so. After a few treatments, it was old news. I'd walk in, climb on the table, take my shirt and bra off, and zone out for a few minutes. Then the clothes would go back on, and we'd be off to another appointment. It was nice to be treated with something that didn't hurt. Radiation didn't cut. It didn't make me sick. And it didn't start to burn until almost the end.

When the sores finally did start appearing, they were more of a nuisance than actually painful. They lined my throat and the back of my mouth, making eating, drinking, and just plain swallowing difficult. The worst part about the sores was the medicine they gave me to help them. That stuff tasted like orange cough syrup stirred into a solution made from car tires. I love how doctors put fruit flavor in something and suddenly it was not supposed to be a big deal anymore. "It's OK! It's fruit flavored!" *Oh, well in that case, I'll take two!* But I was on to them. Cherry flavor didn't help with baby aspirin, and orange flavor didn't help with any of the stuff they were giving me now.

This was my new life, and it became routine surprisingly fast.

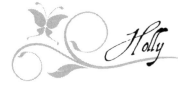

Holly

The memory that will forever stick in my head was when Lindsey lost the majority of her hair for the first time. I was spending the night at her house, and her mom made her go take a shower before bed. She had been losing some hair here and there, but not a ton. When she got out of the shower, she put on a nightgown and came into the living room so Linda could brush her hair. She was sitting on the couch, and I was sitting in a chair facing her. Lindsey sat down on the floor in front of Linda, who started trying to brush the tangles out of her long, wet, light brown, wavy hair. But every time she brushed, she pulled all the hair out with the brush. The brush never got through Lindsey's hair, it just grabbed it all and lifted it off in clumps. Her mom got this look of shock and panic in her eyes, and then shot me a look like, Don't you dare freak out. Play it cool, nothing's wrong, don't scare her. *I think she hid the pile of hair from Lindsey behind her back or somewhere else out of sight. I tried as hard as I could to act like everything was fine, but I was completely stunned and thought to myself,* OK, here we go, now this is real, I can see it.

Linda

I had to go to the school to talk to the principal and the staff, and even any parents who had misunderstandings about cancer actually being contagious. Again, we were dealing with erroneous information, emotional reactions, and rumors. I had to get everyone on the same page. I outlined the treatment protocol. I talked about what kinds of side effects they might see. We decided how to handle homework assignments. They took an "It's OK, don't worry about it, we'll make it happen" approach. I think this was a big benefit of sending Lindsey to a small private school. Yes, we could have pulled her out of school and home schooled her, but I thought it was important for her overall well-being to have a social connection. I wanted her to be able to come to school and be a kid when she wasn't at home feeling sick. I remember the doctors feeling that way, too. Every time she could go back to school after treatments, I volunteered in the classroom so I could watch her and make sure she wasn't too tired or too sick.

We had to put an announcement in the school bulletin advising parents to keep their kids home if they thought they had been exposed to chicken pox. We had to know if there was a chicken pox risk so we could pull her out of school. Chicken pox was potentially deadly, and the risk for severe shingles was high, even though she'd had already it before.

I went half days to school at first, a couple weeks after I came home from surgery—as soon as I could reliably walk without hurting myself and had weaned myself off the support blanket. I was slightly thinner than before, but otherwise I still looked like everyone else. I had some special privileges, like being able to keep some food in my desk. Nothing good. Just Saltines. Since I hated food so much of the time, everyone thought it should be available in case I fancied something, anything. The general rule was, "If she thinks she might want to eat it, give it to her." Dr. Wolff had warned us about chicken pox, and a letter had gone out to all the parents in the school instructing them to inform the office immediately if any child had been exposed to the virus. I had chicken pox when I was five. Somehow, even though I had the antibodies, I could get it again and it could kill me. *Kill me?* I'm not sure I actually believed that. The biggest problem with this idea was that my brother, Travis, had yet to get the disease, and if he were exposed, one of us would have to move out for the virus's incubation period and then some—about 3 weeks. Papa was also a concern. He had a history of shingles, so to be on the safe side, I wasn't supposed to get too chummy with him, either.

On the eighteenth day after my first dose of chemo, I noticed hair on my pillow. When I showered, it got stuck in the tape that still held my incision shut. I spent a fair amount of each day picking it out. My hairbrush was more like a hair harvester. It was funny how it fell out. It was never systematic, always in clumps. I was left with sparse, patchy, scraggly wisps. Mom wanted to make sure I was comfortable with being bald, so she invested in a human hair wig–and I do mean invest. Those suckers cost hundreds of dollars. She found a place in Portland that made them and took me to get fitted. We ordered a dark brown, shoulder-length wig. The woman showed us how to wrap this pink tape around the crown of my head and secure the wig to the tape.

Mind you, because all of my hair was falling out—brows, lashes, arms, etc.—I thought that the wig looked weird. Plus, it was also very heavy and always wanted to slide backward. No one else really seemed to notice, however (or they were too polite to say anything), and if I suddenly appeared without the wig, people would freak out—never to me, of course, always to my parents or friends. Holly would stand up for me by freaking people out right back. Classmates would come up to her, asking quietly what happened to my hair. She'd say, "Oh, you want to know where her hair went? She sneezed, OK? She sneezed and it flew right off her head. She doesn't like to talk about it, either, so don't ask." In the end, the wig fell by the wayside, except for important events where Mom thought it more appropriate for me to wear hair rather than freak people out. I favored my growing collection of crazy caps. I found hats covered in rhinestones, sequins, buttons, and pearls. Hypercolor hats, denim hats, and hats made of satin. I had golf caps, berets, bowlers, stocking caps, and straw hats. A hat for any mood. Of course, if I was feeling bad, spiteful, or lazy, I just wouldn't wear a hat at all. Sometimes, it could be satisfying to see other people wig out.

I would disappear from school for days or weeks at a time. Holly was the main source of information for my peers. If I hadn't turned up in a while, they went to her. Some days I was home with mouth sores from radiation. Sometimes, I was throwing up. Some days I had mouth sores *and* was throwing up; it stung something pretty. Sometimes, my blood counts were too marginal and I didn't have enough energy or immunity to face school. Some days I was having a procedure, radiation, getting chemo, or simply at a clinic appointment.

I'd hear that the kids would wonder what it all meant. Holly herself asked our principal, Sister Mary, "Why is this happening to her?" Sister replied, "God is testing her." I remember Holly telling me that she got angry at her for saying that. I thought, *At least the Catholics don't buy that whole God-is-punishing-you-for-the-sins-of-your-ancestors thing anymore.* But still, what was that supposed to mean anyway? *God is testing her.* OK. So? If I die, did that mean I failed His test? Or did it mean I passed the test and was rewarded with eternity in heaven? Or did it mean that God was suddenly done testing me and had decided to test my family? And what if I lived? Did God give me a gold star?

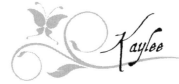

Kaylee

I had just started working in peds oncology. My first memory is learning all the information they got after they scanned her. We knew all that they'd seen and I thought, "She's gonna die. Damn. They're such a nice, perfect family. She's such a nice young girl." I looked at her age, and then when I learned she had mets in her lungs, that's how I knew. Because I'd been taking care of another girl who had almost the same situation and she died. So I prepared myself as best as I could, knowing that that is where we were headed. After awhile of working in that environment, you just are always prepared for things to not be right. I kept waiting for a treatment to not work, for something else to go wrong.

Life on chemo is a very peculiar thing. At least I was too young to have seen any movies or read any books about cancer, so I had no expectations. As they told us in the beginning, people react very differently to chemo. Some don't lose their hair. Some don't throw up. Some people's hair grows back very differently—curly instead of straight or dark brown instead of blond. But everyone suffers the immunity problems—what the docs called "myelosuppression." They said that's how we knew the chemo was working. As I learned more about what myelosuppression entailed, I lowered my expectations for myself. I wouldn't be strong enough to ride my horse. I wouldn't be safe enough from cooties to go to school. But Dr. Wolff wanted me to stay on normal schedules and said it was all about what my priorities were. He told a story about a patient of his who loved playing football so much that no matter how tired or sick he was, he went to practice every day. I thought, *Wolffy, you're crazy, man, if you think I can go off and run like that. I can hardly go up a flight of stairs without stopping for a rest.*

The most disconcerting side effects concerned smells and tastes. Everywhere I went a smell was either comforting or disgusting—usually the latter. I became intolerant of my favorite foods: pizza was too acidic to stay down, ice cream came right back up—more quickly if I ate it too fast. Similarly, the smell of coffee was truly abhorrent; the worst part was that the entire hospital complex was thickly permeated with its odor. I would try and hold my breath as long as possible when walking through the hallways at the clinic. Even if I breathed through my mouth, it was almost as though I could taste it. I remembered reading in school that dogs have a sense of smell several hundred times greater than ours. I wondered if Sassy hated the stink of coffee. Probably not. She liked to roll in dead things.

Consequently, various smells kept me feeling nauseous a lot. I couldn't keep food down, much less the antibiotics—everyone always referred to them as "horse pills" but they looked more like river rock sized pills to me. I will always remember the label on the bottle of pills: *sulfamethoxazole: take 1 pill in the morning and 1/2 in the evening for three days out of the seven.* We had tried every which way to Sunday of getting and keeping those pills down. I wasn't good at swallowing pills anyway, and it was a slippery slope. We tried cutting them in half, but I gagged. Then into fourths, but that didn't work out very well either. Then we cut them down to eighths. Still my gag reflex would win over. If I could get seven down but couldn't get the eighth down, the taste of the errant pill would bring all the others back up and I'd have to start over. Dad would often sit at the table with me the whole time, trying to coach me through it. We tried taking them with thicker milk. Even then, the pill might slowly go down sideways and come straight back up. We tried grinding them up and stirring the powder into yogurt—awful. Pudding was a little better. Mom would get fed up with it all and tell me to "get a grip." I dared her to lick one.

The good news about all this was that because I was dropping weight, they said that when it came to food, all bets are off. I could eat anything I wanted when I wanted if I thought it would stay down. Kudos bars became a favorite, as did dry cereal and Dr. Pepper. Of course, bland things like buttered toast and chicken broth were standbys, but who'd take that over a nice, fat Kudos? I wouldn't. Unless the chocolate reappeared. Which it sometimes did.

One of the biggest problems with food was that if I went long enough without it, I flat out wasn't interested anymore, even though I knew a piece of toast would make me feel infinitely better. If Mom couldn't force it down, I'd end up vomiting as a result of acidic unrest in the tum-tum. This would start a vicious cycle that led to dehydration. One incident in particular involved dropping roughly fifteen pounds over one weekend from vomiting and not being able to keep any water or food down. First thing Monday morning, Dr. Wolff brought me in for IV fluids, and pow! Problem solved.

PART ONE: The Cancer

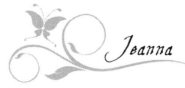

Jeanna

Not long after Lindsey returned from the hospital, I remember her kneeling on the chair in her parents' tiny kitchen, trying to eat some cereal. Her hair was almost gone, and her skin was gray. It took my breath away. I'd been through all of this with them to this point, read the information, talked to the doctors, and I should've expected it, because I knew what it was going to do. But it caught me completely off guard.

I woke up in the middle of the night once with a strange feeling on one side of my face. I swiped my cheek with one hand and felt like I'd removed some snot. *Great, another cold.* I turned over and sniffed. But it kept running. I kept sniffing. I wiped my nose again with my hand, and this time I noticed it didn't feel quite like snot. It wasn't quite slippery. It was almost sticky. I turned on the light. My pillow was covered in a large pool of dark brown blood. I put my hand to my face. Blood. Horrified, I jumped up and went to the mirror, gasping when I saw myself. Part of one half of my face and most of my upper lip and mouth were covered in blood. Thankfully, none had managed to get on my nightgown.

Mom heard me rustling around through the baby monitor—they had installed one when I came home from surgery in case I needed help—and came running in. She didn't seem surprised but just went about helping clean me up. We stopped the nosebleed and she changed out the pillow and we both went back to sleep. That kind of thing was just par for the cancer course. After a few of them, I didn't even mark it as significant anymore. I'd wake up, recognize the symptoms, and think, *Hmm, another bloody nose.* I'd pinch it. It'd stop after a while, and I'd go back to sleep.

Other nights I was clenched with nausea, and I always slept with a chunder chalice next to the bed. Sometimes, in that place between asleep and awake, I would moan and toss restlessly, feeling sick. Soon, Mom or Dad would wake me up, having heard me on the baby monitor. Often, it was enough for one of them to stroke my forehead until I fell back asleep. Occasionally, Mom or

Dad would squeeze into bed with me, and though cramped, I'd fall asleep easily.

I missed ninety-three and one half days of school that year. Spending all that time in the clinic getting chemo or fluids, at home vomiting, or too tired to go anywhere became pretty depressing. When I felt strong enough, I would go spend time with my horse, Misty, grooming her or going out on a trail ride, and that was a major upper. Some days she was too strong for me, which was saying a lot since she was a swaybacked old steed, and that was a major downer. Other days I simply opted to stay at home.

I had a comfortable daily routine. Around eight or nine o'clock, I would wake up. Travis and Mom would be at school and work. Since it was winter, Dad would either be at home or across the street at the shop, fixing equipment or planning for spring planting. Mornings generally were pretty good. Since cereal was one of the foods that worked for me, I didn't pass it up. I would spend an hour or two reading, or doing homework. Mostly, though, I drew pictures. I loved to draw pictures–usually of horses. That was, by and large, how I whiled away the long hours. But I also had a specific TV schedule. We didn't have cable, so I would switch between the four local affiliate stations, depending on what was on. At eleven a.m., it was *Highway to Heaven*. At noon, Dad would come home to check on me and have lunch. *Perry Mason* would be on, which I only watched because Dad liked it so much. It was black-and-white and boring. One p.m. brought *Matlock,* which I loved—he always solved the case just in time in his periwinkle suit!—followed at two by *Hawaii Five-O*—"Book 'em, Danno!" Tedium was overcome at three p.m. when weekday cartoons came on, and soon after, to my delight, everyone was home again.

One evening, Dad was left in charge of me while Mom and Travis were out doing something else. I had woken up from a long nap that afternoon, and Mom had left a note instructing Dad to feed me *something* even if didn't want it. I told him I wasn't hungry.

"Come on," he cooed, drawing out the O's, "there has to be something here we could get for you." In another life, he might be trying to twirl a piece of my hair as he coaxed me to eat. But there was no hair.

He then proceeded to go through the freezer, fridge, cupboards, and drawers, naming their contents and seeking something I could agree to. Turns out, there was a Boboli crust in the fridge. I perked, "OK. I'll eat some pizza."

"You want pizza?" He paused, eyeing it, as if assessing its mastery level. "Yeah, I guess we could figure that out." Twenty minutes later, a mini pizza was sitting in front of me. It smelled great. I slowly at one piece. It tasted great. I went into a feeding frenzy and wolfed the rest down before the mood could pass. It was a little mini heaven.

Afterward, Dad came out with the Septra. We'd switched from the pill form to the liquid in hopes that it wouldn't be quite so vile. I swear the bottle was at least one liter, and I had to get down three tablespoons. There were three available flavors: grape, cherry, and orange. Not wanting grape Septra to ruin Dimetapp for me, I voted for cherry—the token flavor for liquid meds. Three tablespoons. I couldn't decide what was worse: eight tiny little jagged pills or three shovelfuls of liquid. I choked it down, gagging.

People always say, "Hold your nose and it won't taste so bad." That is totally not true. Afterward, we retired to the living room to watch *America's Funniest Home Videos*, with the goal of keeping the septra down for a minimum of 40 minutes. Immediately my tumtum was unhappy. We barely had enough time to get through the show's opening credits before the Boboli made a reappearance. As I was throwing up so hard that some of the contents dripped from my nose, I noted that the second showing of the Boboli was more palatable than the cherry flavored Septra. But that was the last I saw of a Boboli for a *very* long while.

Dad took care of the vomit, and we started over again with the meds.

With patterns like these, it didn't take long for me to go from my original 120 pounds to the upper 90s or low 100s. My nadir was eighty-nine. Accompanying a frequently empty stomach and dropping thirty pounds is cold. Perpetual, numbing cold. Fortunately, it wasn't the seizing and shivering cold that is a result of fevers or infection, but rather a low-grade consistent chill—especially in my hands and feet. This would be compounded by the fact that my mother was a compulsive house-airer. Whenever she would clean, she'd open the windows and doors for twenty minutes—even in the dead of winter!—to air out the house. My protesting was useless. If my attempts to warm myself with half a dozen blankets or a lapdog failed, I'd head to the shower. I often would feel too tired to stand in the shower for a long time, so it became my routine to turn on the shower as hot as I could stand and lay down in the tub, letting the warm water fall on me. I could almost fall asleep in the shower. I would have, I'm sure, if I wasn't afraid that the warm water would run out while I was sleeping and I'd end up just as cold as before. The burning sensation of hot water on cold skin became pleasurable and comforting because I knew it was the only thing that would make me feel better. Over time, I developed a massive appreciation for showers as hot as I could comfortably stand. When I felt the water temperature start to wane, I'd tap the lever with my foot to warm it up, until all the hot water had been used up. Generally, it would take between forty minutes and an hour. Since I didn't have wet hair to worry about, I could stay warm really well if I dried off quickly, bundled up in pants and socks and a hat, and jumped back under all the blankets. Bonus points if the dog was still there warming my place.

Aside from just not eating, and feeling like I was standing naked outside in Siberia, some of the strangest experiences of my life, to date, were being mistaken for a boy by strangers and passersby. Sometimes, people were simply making polite observations about "what a darling boy" my mother had. Mom didn't try to correct them. It probably would have been more embarrassing for them anyway. Other times, I wondered at how stupid they really were. For instance, I had an outfit, which I called my 101 Dalmatians outfit—white pants with big black polka dots and a matching shirt. I would pair this with one of my aforementioned caps, perhaps with a *pink* one or one covered in *rhinestones*. And yet, these people would look at me, examine my ensemble, raise their eyebrows, and smiling all the while a smile that was freakishly large, they would exclaim, "My, what an interesting outfit for a little boy." I didn't realize until years later that they probably thought I might be the youngest gay boy to come out. Most of the time I shrugged it off. It never really made me angry that they were so ignorant, but I would wonder how they could overlook the fact that I was a little too pale and a little too bald to be a regular eleven-year-old boy.

I never brooded upon these comparisons until one day I was at Holly's house, and we decided to go play in the front yard. Holly lived on the major thoroughfare through the city of Forest Grove, a few blocks from Pacific University. As we dashed through the front door and down the porch steps, I paused, realizing I'd forgotten my hat. I didn't care enough to go back for it. Just then, a black Toyota 4Runner loaded with college boys slowed and stopped at the red light at the intersection in front of her house. They were watching us, laughing and chattering to each other, but I was oblivious until the driver yelled out the window, "God, who'd ever want to date *you*?" This was followed by peals of laughter from everyone else in the car. At first, I didn't realize they were addressing me. As it slowly dawned on me, I couldn't understand why someone would want to say something like that. Surely, seeing a skinny kid with no hair or eyebrows was enough information for someone to think, *Oh, maybe that kid has cancer.* I mean, it's not exactly a secret, what we look like. I continued to watch them. The light turned green, and they started to drive off. As I turned to go back into the shadows of the house, I heard Holly scream out behind me, "Hey, *fuck you,* assholes!" I smiled. She fixed *their* wagon.

The sound of the car and the laughter faded out behind the latching front door, and I realized it was my own fault I had been made fun of. I'd never go outside without a cap again. Later, Holly and I decided that anyone that stupid didn't belong in college anyway.

In retrospect, being eleven at the time of such an insult was serendipitous. Boys occupied very little time on my radar anyway, and consequently, I suffered very little self-esteem problems concerning whether or not I was date-able. But the problem didn't close with the front door that afternoon. The issue of whether or not I could be pretty after something like this would again raise itself years later, as I began dating in high school and college.

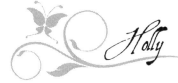

The only way I knew how to help was to be there. I came from a family that deals with tragedy by joking about things to make us feel lighter and forget the drama and pain, if only for a few minutes. So, I did just that. I mercilessly needled Dr. Wolff (Wolffy!), just being the absolute sassiest thing on the planet towards him. Maybe that was my way of taking back power from him. He wasn't such a scary, serious cancer doctor if I could make fun of him and get on his nerves. What a brat I was.

Putting surgical masks on our heads to look like Mennonite women. Wheelchair races. Looking over the nurse's shoulder when she unlocked the movie closet so I could break in with the combination and get movies whenever Lindsey wanted one. I still think the combination was 12354. Buying Lindsey really ugly baseball caps to wear. She had that big box of them in the right side of her closet. Oh, God, denim with rhinestones! Hot pink with a bow! So nineties!

Dr. Wolff would call occasionally to check in or announce lab results. I could tell he didn't like to talk on the phone very much. He always greeted you with a quick, "Yeah, it's Dr. Wolff." Then you'd talk about whatever he called about, and he would never say good-bye. He always said something like, "Catch ya later," or "See you soon," or even just a "Yeah. Uh-huh." Mom thought he never said good-bye because he had to work so closely with children who could die quickly and easily.

I might be up at the clinic as often as three times a week, excluding extra trips if I couldn't stop vomiting or needed fluids. You get very close to the people who are caring for you when you spend that much time with them. Dr. Wolff was my absolute favorite. Sometimes, if he was gone, Dr. Norman would be in charge, which was also great. That man was an absolute scream.

One time, Mom and I were up because I couldn't manage to dispel my nausea with the Reglan and Benadryl, and I'd taken so much that I wasn't really sleeping it off, either. Both Wolff and

Norman were out of the clinic that day, which left Dr. Stein. I still always thought of her as "the woman with the ear cuffs." She was very abrupt. Dr. Wolff could be abrupt, too, but I actually liked him, so it was OK. Dr. Stein just wasn't for me. She came into the exam room that day, where I was curled up on the table, and asked my mom what the "deal" was. When Mom explained, Stein walked over and bent down, looking right in my face. She was close-talking me. "You can puke now, or you can puke later. Those are the options." With not so much as a "Sorry, kid, that's just the way the cookie crumbles," she was gone. In her defense, there was nothing she could have done anyway. This was the dark age before the miracle of antinausea drugs.

To my vast surprise, the radiation oncologists stopped therapy much sooner than they expected. After little more than two weeks, the chest X-ray showed that all the lesions in my lungs were undetectable. They stopped treatment. That was fine with me, seeing as how by then I had plenty of sores in my throat and mouth and was drinking the orange/rubber cocktail too often for my taste.

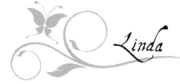

The worst thing, by far, was trying to get blood out of her. She would have major meltdowns each and every time. And the more she tensed up, the worse it became to try and get blood out. It was always hard to find someone who could successfully butterfly her. Kaylee was pretty good at it. It takes a special finesse and dynamic with Lindsey to have a successful blood draw. If Kaylee couldn't do it, Wolff could.

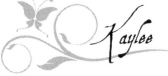

Lindsey had incredible anxiety about getting labs drawn. Back then, there wasn't any program in place to help mitigate that, so she was just totally freaked out, out of control, and irrational. And of course this provokes anxiety in me as a caregiver. I absolutely had to be perfect about getting a draw. But you're doomed because the physiological anxiety response is destroying your ability to actually hit a vein. And you could see it start as soon as she walked in the room. She would get this look on her face, and her skin would pale. It was horrible to watch, this poor young lady, who otherwise was such a pleasure to take care of. As I would try to stabilize her arm for the actual poke, she'd pull against me and start to cry, sometimes hyperventilating. I recall trying to rationalize with her, but there wasn't anything I could say or do to change any of it. The look in her eyes was just so...she couldn't even engage with me. She was just on a whole different planet.

When it came time for the Adriamycin (doxorubicin) and actinomycin (dactinomycin) treatments, instead of being pushed through the butterfly all at once, they were given over three and five days, respectively, and required much more work. I would show up, and they would call IV therapy. Someone who "specialized" in starting IVs would show up an hour later, and the endless struggle to find my pipelines would begin. Usually, we'd run out of time before they could find a viable vein, and they'd have to leave for their next appointment. Or if it was a really good day, they'd find a vein, secure the IV, and leave just in time for the vein to collapse and render the IV useless. Trying to find a way to pump up my veins, mom brought home a stress-ball for me, but even it failed us. Eventually we gave up on IV therapy. and Dr. Wolff would just roll up his sleeves and put in the butterfly himself. Then he taped my arm to a board and covered it in this sleeve-like glove. Wolff was a pro at finding veins. He was trained in an era when finding and hitting children's tiny veins was one of the most important skills a pediatrician could have—there were no central lines back in those days. He told me once that he had a number of patients who started their own IVs. He said this in a suggestive way, as if I might want to try it. I thought that was crazy, and told him so. He just slowly shrugged at me, as if to say, "OK. Your choice."

Once they got the butterfly in, they'd hook the tube up to the IV and away we went. There would be an hour of plain old saline fluids first; then Patsy or Kaylee would come in and inject the giant syringe of chemo into the IV drip. Adriamycin was a deep, powerful red. When it diluted and flowed through the line, it turned an orange color. Patsy came in once while I was staring at the orange line creeping ever toward my arm and said, "It looks a lot like Orange Crush, doesn't it?" So it did. Then I wondered what it would feel like to put Orange Crush in my veins, to feel the carbonation prickling underneath my skin, and I felt suddenly sick.

Once the drip was going, there was nothing to do but wait it out, which we usually did with homework, magazines or a sketch pad. One day, we were sitting around feeling exceptionally bored when Mom suddenly piped up with, "Let's write a poem!" Oh, of course. A poem. "Let's write one about Dr. Wolff!" she exclaimed. I wasn't sure about that. I didn't know if Dr. Wolff would *want* such a poem, but she was on a roll. "Let's call it 'The Bow Tie Being.' What do you think?" she asked, beaming. Thinking she'd just said "Bow Tie Bean" I laughed uncontrollably. How did she come up with this stuff? Mom began to compose out loud, chewing on the cap of her pen. "Hmm...How about 'Come one, come all! This is worth seeing.'" She paused, thinking. "More than we can count... it's the Bow Tie Being!" We both giggled, decided it was a keeper, and scribbled it down.

"What color bow tie should we write about?" I asked, now interested in this project. I liked his red tie best. Mom liked the yellow.

"Hmm...how about 'You can gauge his mood by the color he wears.'" She wrote as she recited. "'Red is to be feared, 'cause you're worried...'" she trailed off, thinking. "You're worried... hmm, what should we be worried about?" she asked, looking up at me. We were quiet, thinking how best to end such a profound stanza. Then I had a brilliant idea.

"Oh, I know! 'Because you're worried he swears'!" I shouted, clapping my hands. We rolled in hysterics for a few minutes before regaining enough control to plow forward with our poetry. The next stanza was devoted to the yellow tie. When we had decided on the wording, I read her notes out loud, "Yellow is our favorite. It's warm and vibrant tones show off the Being's smile as he jokes on the phone." From there, the creative juices flowed. By the time we were done composing, we were wiping tears from our eyes, and our stomachs hurt from laughing so hard. I rewrote the notes into a proper poem in my best cursive. When we saw him later that afternoon, I handed over the poem and watched anxiously while he read it, grinning and shaking his head.

"I'm going to keep this in my office," he announced with a smile.

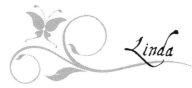

Linda

We were part of a study. Some people were assigned fifteen months of treatment, and some people got six months. We got six. Shortly after we finished treatment, the study was eventually published saying that the six months of treatment was as effective as fifteen months in preventing relapse. I was so glad. I had been worried that we weren't doing the right thing, that six months wouldn't be enough.

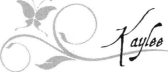

Kaylee

I for some reason always tend to think the worst with all the patients. Maybe it was a coping mechanism for me. So at the end of her treatment, I was thinking to myself, don't get too excited. She's not going to be out there for very long. *It's a sad thing to say that back in those days the mentality was just* OK, you're done. Go live your life. Good luck getting insurance someday. Good luck dealing with all those secondary side effects. *It just wasn't thought about so much then. I certainly didn't think of it then.*

After what felt like an eternity of pill-popping, countless collapsed veins, dozens of incompetent IV therapists and hardly a week gone by without at least one episode of vomiting, it was May 10, 1992.

The Moment of Truth.

I had completed my last chemotherapy cycle and was in for a draw and a checkup. It was sunny that day. Dr. Wolff came in again with the huge binder—presumably the same one we'd seen on our first day in the clinic—and that was significant because the man almost never carried files with him. He essentially never took notes during a physical exam, and he didn't need to because his recall was impeccable. I would marvel at how he could remember so many miniscule details about me just off the top of his head. That day, however, he was referring to the notes about the Wilms Tumor study, and that meant it was an important day. But I wasn't listening to what he was saying. I was on pins and needles. My heart was racing. My hands were clammy. Would I go home for good? Would I stay for more? The thought of being assigned to another nine months of chemo was horribly depressing. What would I do? How could I stand nine more months? That was…270 days! I would still be on treatment when I started the seventh grade in September. If he came back in and the verdict was nine more months, I might start shrieking.

I couldn't think about that.

My heart was going a mile a minute. I squirmed on the exam table while Dr. Wolff looked in my ears, nose, eyes, and mouth. I always had to stifle a laugh when he looked at my eyes, because he got so close with the scope, and his one eye was all squinted shut so that it looked like his head was a really weird shape. Like I was seeing through a convex lens. He rubbed the bell of the stethoscope briskly on his hands and pressed it to my back to listen to me breathe. After going to the front to hear the ol' ticker, he said, "Lie down and bend your knees a little, please and thank you." I did. He always said "please and thank you," I thought, smiling inwardly. He pushed up my shirt to examine the op site. The incision was a dull dark pink and as pencil-thin as ever. When his hands moved over the now nerveless skin, I felt only pressure. I was tense and restless. He stopped prodding for a second. "Hey. Where's the fire?" he asked incredulously. "You have a pressing appointment today? Can you just hold still for two seconds?" When he finished, I shot back up to a sitting position. He looked at the ceiling, thinking. Then he rubbed his eyes, as he always did when he was thinking, planning.

"Ah…OK, I'm going to go check the computer. Give me a few minutes." He swept from the door of the exam room and closed it behind him. Neither Mom nor I said a word. The minutes ticked by like centuries. I couldn't stop thinking about it. What would be the result? How great would it be to be free today? But that won't happen, I just know it. We're going to get the 15 month protocol. Oh, that will be awful. I oscillated back and forth with these thoughts until he came back, sporting his signature broad Wolffy grin.

"Go home. Get outta here."

"We're through?" Mom asked. I stared with my mouth hanging open. This sounded too good to be true.

"We still need to watch you," he said to me. "Talk to Kaylee about seeing you later in the week. But treatment's through."

Oh my God. I was going home! My hair would grow back! I'd be able to ride my horse again…run…play…whatever. *It was over.*

The weekly visits to Dr. Wolff's office turned into bimonthly visits, then monthly, and eventually quarterly. My hair started to grow back, thick and dark, and pin curly—just like everyone said it might. By November of 1992, when school pictures were taken again, I had a total Afro. Dad used to say, "Don't bother wearing a helmet when you ride your horse. If you fall, you'll just spring back up on your hair." My aversions to coffee, pizza, ice cream, and all other foods that had elicited a hearty barf in the last six months faded. I got my strength back, my wind, and eventually my weight. In October, I turned twelve, and it was a very big deal. From that point on, celebrating another year of life in our family was always a big deal. Everything was going back to normal.

Including my biological clock, it seemed. About eight months after I finished treatment, I got my first period. For real, this time. I had a momentary flashback to that nightmarish afternoon when we'd been fooled by the cancer before gathering my wits and going about the necessary business. This was just another mark of normalcy.

For the next fifteen months, life went on as it had before. I went to school. I galloped my horse. I started wearing makeup. And I forgot much about what had happened, aside from seeing Dr. Wolff every once in awhile.

It was a normalcy that would be short-lived.

I was accompanying my cousins on a camping trip in Central Oregon when my dad was nearly killed on the farm.

The farm uses high-pressure irrigation systems, a way to water large swaths of a field at one time. Such systems are very common-place now, but there were many ways for things to go wrong and people to get hurt. In short, it is a very giant sprinkler that rolls its way through the fields. Simply, the system draws water from the river with one pump at the waterline that sends it up to a "booster" pump at the top of the bank. That pump sends the water out to the pipeline. It's the second pump that brings the pressure up to about 200psi. The water flies through hundreds or thousands of feet of six-inch diameter galvanized aluminum pipe and black rubber hose—much bigger and more durable than a firefighter's hose—to an irrigation "gun" that shoots about a two-hundred-foot arc across the field.

Early one morning, Dad was out to move the gun to a different part of the field, and was taking apart some pipe. The first rule of farming is to never let yourself be distracted from what you're doing. That's the quickest, easiest way to get hurt. The second rule is never stand in front of an object that could detach from the pipe and shoot out. One such object is called an end-plug, which is used to block water flow from one end of a T-pipe. Dad broke both rules simultaneously.

So there he was, at seven a.m. on a bright August morning, standing in front of the end plug as he pried it off its pipe. Now, after turning off the water, it takes awhile for the pipes to drain the water and release all the pent-up air. The air pressure in the system had not yet bled out, and the plug shot off the pipe, nailed his leg, and flew out into the cornfield. It tore off his shoe and knocked him down. When he dared look, the pipe was draining river water everywhere, and his leg was cracked open and bleeding. He could see the splinters of what remained of his ankle joint. He thought,

People always say when you're injured like this, it doesn't hurt. But this hurts like hell! He panicked for a second, as he lay there in the mud and running river water. Gathering his wits, he weighed his options. He was roughly a mile from the farmhouse. It's seven o'clock in the morning. This was the era before cell phones were common. Nobody would even begin to wonder where he was until after dark that night. His leg was broken. Badly. If he lay out there and waited for help, he'd likely die of shock.

A few yards away sat the Honda ATV that we used to flit from field to field on the property. He dragged himself through the mud and water, hoisted himself up on the four-wheeler, draping his broken leg over his arm on the handlebar, and slowly, carefully putted to the house. They called an ambulance, and within hours Dad was in surgery to reconstruct what his surgeons called a "war wound the likes of which [they'd] only seen in textbooks."

Later, Dad's brother was walking through the field to finish what Dad had started that morning, and he found the end plug some forty feet from the pipe to which it had been attached. The impact had made a large dent and stripped the galvanization. He also found the shoe, and the laces were ripped in half.

I heard this whole story during the car ride from my house, where my cousins had just dropped me off, to the hospital where Dad was in Intensive Care. This was only the beginning of what was in store for the VanDykes in the winter of 1993.

Linda

The time off from cancer had been great. Things never went back to "normal" 100 percent, because Lindsey had to get to a two-year mark before she could be considered "cured." What is "normal" anyway after you've been diagnosed? Nothing goes back to normal once you've been diagnosed, so you just develop a new normal. But in the meantime, we didn't have to worry about it or think about it. Always hated having to go in and have checkups, though. I would get worried at the checkups.

Just before the first day of my eighth-grade year, we were at the peds hem/onc clinic for the usual battery of tests: blood draw, physical, chest X-ray. They would run a very fine-toothed comb over me during these checkups. Wolff carefully looked over every inch of my body: lymph nodes, legs, abdomen, lungs, eyes, spine, everything. It all went well, and at the end of the day my films were sent to a board of radiologists, as usual, for inspection. One doctor out of the whole group caught the tiniest hint of a shadow on the upper part of my right lung. We received a call from Dr. Wolff.

"We need you to come up for a CT as soon as you can."

"Why?" Mom asked. "What happened?"

"It seems that one of the radiologists on the board thought she saw something, so I want to order a CT just so we can cover all our bases." So it was a casual thing. Just go up, do the scan, nothing to worry about, we're just double-checking. No big deal. The first day of school was a half day, so we scheduled to come up at noon.

Mom and Dad picked Travis and me up from school, and away we went. Whenever I was scheduled for a test outside of the peds hem/onc clinic, Wolff always had me check in with him first. Good thing, because almost without fail, CT was in a different place every time due to new construction. When we finally got there, we had to wait for a long time, and then a technician came back and called for me. The routine was always the same: drink this, take that off, put this on, do that, have a blanket, hold still, breathe in, breathe out, don't move, time for the contrast, just awhile longer, now we're done, wait for the films, they'll be right out. Those guys in CT always took forever. When they finally came out and handed me the oversize envelope, we slowly picked our way through buildings and wings until we found the clinic again.

All the exam rooms were full, but the waiting room was dead empty and there were no more appointments for the day, so Patsy took the films and told us to go out there. Travis drew on the chalkboard and played with all the toys while Mom, Dad, and I sat around in the child-sized chairs and waited in the navy blue room.

Dr. Wolff appeared after some time. "Well, hey there, Travis, what have you got there?"

"Super NES. It's *Mario Kart*," Travis said, without looking away from the screen. Wolff slowly shook his head at him, grinning.

"That stuff's beyond me." He stopped for a second. "It's amazing. He really looks like a young Paul McCartney." We looked. Three heads in unison. None of us had ever made that connection, but Dr. Wolff was right. The perfectly arched eyebrows, long lashes on big brown eyes, the boyish nose, and the perfect mouth. Sure enough, an eight-year-old version of that famous Liverpudlian was in our midst.

Dr. Wolff rubbed his eyes and continued, "Ah...we should talk. I wish we had a better room than this..." He paused, crossing his arms, and again putting a hand over his eyes, rubbing them and thinking. "We've had a chance to look at the films, Dr. Norman, Dr. Stein and I, and it looks like radiology was right. We can see a small—coin-sized—lesion in the upper quadrant of her right lung."

Dead silence. Travis's controller clicked endlessly; the game bleeped and blooped. None of us moved—except Travis, completely enveloped by *Mario Kart*. We looked up at Dr. Wolff who went on, "It looks as though its position matches exactly one that was there before. It's possible that the radiation therapy was able to shrink it beyond detection but not eliminate it entirely."

Silence. I don't even know what I was thinking. Everything and nothing at the same time. The only thought that cleared my brain was *Oh, so here we go again.*

"What do we do?" Mom asked, ready to take charge.

"Is it widespread like before?" Dad added.

"From the scans, it looks like it's alone. I want to get some blood, though"—I groaned, and his eyes darted to me then back to my parents—"and see what we can see. We will be looking at surgery to remove that lesion."

"Tomorrow?" I asked.

"Oh, no, no. Not tomorrow." He almost laughed then became dead serious again. "But probably in the next week or two."

I wanted to get it out as soon as possible. I didn't like the idea of something in there feeding off of me, getting bigger. But none of it really registered because I felt strangely OK with all of this new information. It was almost like a dream, or as though I were sitting in a theatre watching this scene being performed before me. I kept thinking that in any second Mom would rush in, turn the lights on in my room, and shout, "Get up! Time for school!" I would wake up in my own bed, safe and comfortable and still cancer free. I watched Dr. Wolff finish talking, turn, and leave. There was no sound. I looked right. Mom and Dad were talking. I looked left. Travis was still playing. No sound. So, as soon as a room cleared, Kaylee came to get me, holding the Butterfly Tray, and went after three vials of my blood.

We went home from the X-ray after Dr. Wolff said, "Nope, we don't see anything on there." Then we got a call the next day saying. "Actually, the tumor board sees something on there." That was pretty hard to hear because we were so close to having that clean bill of health. I was in denial, or it was wishful thinking on my part that what they'd seen on the X-ray could have been a shadow on the film. I was really convincing myself that it was just a glitch. It was a blow to hear that there was definitely something we had to go after again.

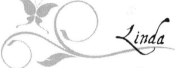

I don't think I even worried about Wes. I knew he would get better. But when Lindsey's diagnosis came down shortly after he had been hurt, I thought, "Are you kidding me? Now we have two people sick?"

Next thing I knew, I was standing in the front yard of our house, watching the sunlight go from gold to red and playing with the dogs. Mom and Dad went into the house with Travis. I stayed outside. I was actually enjoying myself, considering what I had just heard. Denial, perhaps. Sandy Dunes, the little stray mut that had come to live with us a few years before, was up the small pine tree after the starlings. They were teasing her, and pretty soon she couldn't get down. I dragged her out of the tree, and she shot off across the yard after a starling in the grass. She came back and tried to wrestle the pork bone I had for her out of my hands. I threw it. She chased it. For a while, I forgot everything.

I walked into the living room. Mom beeped off the phone and looked at me. I looked back, we said nothing, and then I proceeded to my room. Fifteen minutes later, I walked back out to the kitchen and saw a car careening up our long gravel driveway. It was a burgundy BMW, the reddish sunlight glinting off the roof, and it was coming at us at about warp nine leaving a rooster tail of orange dust behind it. It was Sharon. For a second, I didn't know why she was here. She came bursting into the kitchen and, as Mom started to cry, enveloped her in a hug. I watched this surreal scene. Sharon looked at me.

"How're you doing, punkin? You OK?" Mom continued to sob loudly. I was overwhelmed by the scene before me and the gravity of what Dr. Wolff had said only ninety minutes before. I had cancer. *Again.* It hadn't killed me last time, but it might now. I had to do it all over again. I started to cry, and they drew me into a group hug.

That was a Tuesday. We decided not to tell anyone yet and give ourselves a chance to absorb it all. Only our immediate family, grandparents, Holly, and Sharon knew what had happened. On Sunday afternoon, people started calling. They had been to church, where the priest had said the morning mass for us. What was strange about it, though, was that it wasn't the same church that my grandparents or I go to. We never did find out how the priest knew before anyone else, but Mom said it as a sign that God knew about us and was going to be hanging around.

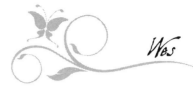

The surgery this time was considerably more invasive. The physical trauma was much more significant the second time around. She was in the ICU after that surgery instead of the regular ward.

At six o'clock in the morning on September 15, 1993, I walked through the same double sliding doors of Doernbecher Children's Hospital through which I had been wheeled twenty-two months before. Checking in, the nurse tied on a yellow wristband with sparkly rainbow colors on it. She sent me up to 14A, where the children's ward was, and the nurse, Karen, put us in a semiprivate room. I made a comment about how when we first came up two years ago, they put us in a quad. She said, "Now that you're thirteen, we try to keep the older kids in semiprivate and private rooms. Younger ones tend to fare better in group environments than the older ones." Karen was very cool. She had long straight hair pulled back in a utilitarian pony; she favored T-shirts and stretch pants and enjoyed rollerblading on the streets of Portland in the middle of the night.

We milled around for a while, while people signed papers, checked that I hadn't eaten anything for twelve hours, and tried to start an IV. I begged them off, asking if they could do it down in surgery. They could. So they left me alone. After another while, the guy in the green coat came with the gurney and one of those magenta gowns. It had snaps up the sleeves—an all-access garment. I remembered the conundrum about what to do with my underwear, but I left them on again. I'd started my period the day before, but I didn't know if this was information anyone needed to know, and they weren't asking. Plus, the idea of lying on my back, fully conscious, and being wheeled around a hospital with no underwear on was too weird. After pulling on the light blue socks with dark blue rubber treads on the sole, I hopped up onto the gurney and we rolled off.

In preop, the anesthesiologist came in. He had a great hat on. He didn't wear one of those mushroom caps but rather a tight-fitting skullcap looking thing. It was dark blue with lots of red chili peppers on it. Did I have any allergies? Did I have an IV yet? Did I know how anesthesia works? Did I know it could make me feel sick afterward and give me a sore throat?

"Yeah, I know how it works. You give me the gas that smells sweet, and I'm out."

"More or less, that's right." He looked at my arms. "We need to start an IV on you."

I went bug-eyed. "Can you do that maybe after I'm asleep?" I asked.

He crossed his arms but not in a defiant way. "Well, we generally like give you a little something here, so you're pretty out of it while we're moving back there. Some people get scared seeing the inside of the operating rooms."

"I won't get scared. I want to remember what it looks like. I think it might be interesting." He looked at me for a second before saying, "OK, sure. If you want." He moved off, and within minutes a flock of masked and gowned individuals surrounded me, and we were off. I lay back and marked our progress by the passing overhead florescent lights. Through the double doors. Around the corner. I leaned up on my elbows, watching. People in mushroom caps turned and stared at me. I thought, *They must not get that many awake people down this way.* Through another door, and there it was, with some more gowned, masked, and gloved people. I saw the chili peppers. This operating room was different than the one I'd seen before. It looked much newer. Everything was white and somehow brighter. They asked me to scoot over onto the table. There were quite a few of those giant dentist lights overhead. More tubing, tanks, shelving, etc. Still no sign of tools, but I didn't look very hard.

"Alrighty," said Chili Peppers, "how about you lay back this way." Reluctantly, I lay down and looked up. They switched the big lights on, positioning them over me. Torsos and masked faces leaned into my field of vision as they did their work. People were bustling around everywhere. I felt like I was in some medical drama. Out of the corner of my eye, I saw a mushroom-capped person maneuvering around my right wrist. I smelled the alcohol and felt the wipe on my skin.

I tensed up.

Everything went rigid as a board. I started breathing hard and fast, noticing my right arm starting to tremble. I felt suddenly sweaty. Before I could even think, I heard Chili Peppers's soothing voice over the din behind me as he put a mask over my face: "OK. Here you go, just breathe this. It's just some laughing gas." I felt someone start feeling around my left arm, too. Then more hands prodding for veins on my feet. One of the men I supposed was a surgeon moved into my field of vision to the left. He had bronze skin and dark, smiling eyes. In a very velvety voice he said, "That stuff always makes me feel like my ears are going to fall off." Oh... my...God...that was *hilarious*! I started to shake with giggles, and pretty soon I couldn't even keep them quiet. They were putting sticky electrodes on my chest. Someone was messing with my arms. Ouch! Son of a...

"We're in!" It came from far away, echoed.

"All right, Lindsey, I'm going to turn on the real stuff. Now, it's going to smell a bit like an old shoe...so give me five good breaths, OK?" OK. Here we went again. I could tell as soon as the new gas crept into my mask. I breathed. One. It had a very unique aroma, not quite like an old shoe, but I suppose that might be a good description. I breathed again. Two. Years later I would use rubber cement in high school art class and have a bit of a brief flashback to the white room full of bustling people, and the feeling of that mask on my face. I breathed again. Three. Darkness descended.

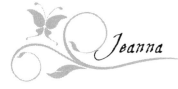

Jeanna

That was a time of my life when everything stopped.

Wes called me and said that they'd found a tiny spot. So tiny. But they wanted to take it out. Couldn't take a risk. My world just went poop! *There were so many bad things that were going on at the same time, with Wes's injury being just one of them. I remember thinking,* Let's just get past all these dark, dark times. This will heal, that will heal, let's just get Lindsey through. *It was like a mantra.*

"Lindsey, can you hear me? If you can hear me, I need you to look at me. Open your eyes." I opened them. They weighed a ton, like a pair of lead-dipped lids. It took all my strength to pry my eyes open and focus on the shape in front of me.

"Do you have any pain?"

"No." *Just let me sleep, lady, please.* I stopped for a second and tested myself for a sore throat or nausea. None. As I fell back into sleepy darkness, I thought, *Who are these chumps that say anesthesia makes you sick and gives you a sore throat... ?*

When I woke again, I was in a strange room. It looked like I was in an aquarium. Mom was there. It was pretty small. Above me and to the right was a monitor, carefully ticking away my pulse, oxygen levels, and blood pressure. In front of me was a TV. To my left was a huge sliding glass door. It was like a little aquarium. It was quiet here. There was a low din from the nurses' station outside my door, but no other noise. I knew from the noise level that we were not on 14A.

"Booie, you know where you are?"

I nodded. "Hospital," I squawked.

"This is intensive care. Look at this thing up here." She pointed to the monitor. "It's watching your air and your heart." She held my right hand up. Taped to the end of my index finger was something like a white clothespin that clamped on. It had a red light on it. "Look, you have an ET finger." The little white cord that came out of the plastic clamp went up to the monitor.

I was uncomfortable. I felt like something was jabbing into my right side of my back. With every breath it jabbed and released, jabbed and released. I squirmed, thinking it wouldn't hurt, thinking that I could rearrange it so it wouldn't jab. How much did you use your upper back muscles anyway, while in bed? Oh, quite a lot, as I soon found out—empirically. Whatever it was that felt like it was jabbing me in the back suddenly exploded with pain, and the rest of my entire right side of my back caught. I hitched a breath—more pain. I tried not to scream, remembering how that had felt the last time. Tears welled up in my eyes and threatened to spill over. I couldn't even breathe this time without pain. *So that's how it's gonna be,* I thought. This time *every* breath would hurt.

Information that might have been useful a few hours ago.

Suddenly, I realized I could hear that same low droning of a motor exactly like before when I had the stomach tube. So they had something sucking stuff out of me again. "You hurt?" Mom asked, almost sternly, ready for battle. I nodded, cringing, tears still pressing against the floodgates. She walked out the door and said something to someone, and a woman came in to ask me what my pain was, from one to ten. God, I was getting sick of that question. *Twelve, people! It's twelve! What's the point of even asking?* I noticed a chart on the wall across from me. For each number a cartoon guy was making a more progressively painful face. At zero, he was smiling contentedly. At ten, he was screaming silently with tears and sweat pouring off his face. I thought, *OK, fine.* So I wasn't a twelve. But I was definitely a healthy eight.

That night, the nurse came in with that old shtick about needing to put an egg crate under the sheet. *Seriously,* I thought, *this has to be a joke.* I'd only just woke up a few hours ago. No joke, this lady wanted me up and in the chair against the wall. I immediately became apprehensive. I'd already figured out that it hurt like hell to take even a deep breath. How was I going to raise myself from the bed without using those vital muscles that had just been severed? Short answer: I wasn't. The nurse put her arm out to brace me and raise me up, but the moment I exerted pressure I could feel the pain ripping through my back, and those things jabbing away with every movement.

"What is *jabbing* me? It hurts!" I declared loudly enough to wake everyone else on the ward. Mom and the nurse looked at me with stupid, puzzled faces.

"Nothing is jabbing you," the nurse said.

"Yes! Right under my ribs back there."

"Oh yeah. Those are chest tubes. I've heard they're pretty uncomfortable, but I've never heard of it as 'jabbing.'"

I scowled at her. "What are they doing in there?"

"They are keeping air pockets from forming between your lung and your chest wall. They're preventing pneumothorax." Pneumothorax. A fancy air bubble was all it amounted to, and yet its prevention was shockingly painful, a tube a couple centimeters in diameter, and not just one. I had *two*.

We started to move. Mom tried to help, but I didn't like anyone with zero medical experience touching me. I don't know how I managed to get from the bed to the chair, but all the while I kept thinking, *There's no way I was in this much pain the last time.* Even if I was, how could I have forgotten it? This had to be the worst pain in the world. I wondered what Dad felt like when he was almost amputated in the field. When I finally collapsed into the chair, it felt like being released from the Rack. As I sat there, watching the nurse strip the bed, unroll the foam pad, and put it in place, something caught my eye to the left. It was the monitor hooked to my ET finger. My heart rate was racing along, like a hummingbird. My blood pressure was skyrocketing. I thought I'd try and experiment and hold my breath. I held it as long as I could, until the burning feeling was no longer bearable. With every second that passed, the heart rate slowed down and the oxygen saturation lines started moving down out of their grid into the one below. Finally I couldn't stand it anymore, and I breathed, ignoring the painful sensation it brought in my back. The oxygen line shot back up into its own grid, and the heart rate increased. How interesting! I wondered if it went low enough whether it would set off an alarm; then I wondered if I could hold my breath long enough to do it.

The nurse's arm thrust into my field of vision and woke me from my reverie. It was time to get up again. I was exhausted and wanted nothing more than to be in that bed sleeping. But how badly did you really want something? If you were dead tired, would it be worth it to you to have someone hammer nails into your body to buy your ticket to some sleep? In my current state of sitting, the only discomfort I felt was a slight tugging from the weight of the chest tubes. How could they make me do this the same day as surgery? At least last time they gave me one night of respite. Come on! I was in Intensive Care, for cryin' out loud! Again, the nurse helped to get me up from the chair, turn around, and sit on the bed. Then she helped me get my feet up and lie down. The worse part was lying down, because I was worried that my arm would give out and I'd fall the extra six or eight inches to the bed, hurting myself even more. The last part was scooting to the middle of the bed and shifting to get comfortable. Very slowly, very gingerly, and not without serious discomfort, I got there. I decided right then that I'd never do anything in my life that could buy myself another surgery like this–no smoking, no huffing glue. I thought if people actually had a clue about how this feels, they'd drop their cigarettes in a heartbeat.

The nurse started to walk out of the room and looked down at something near the foot of my bed, frowning. "Your catheter hasn't drawn anything, yet. That's odd." Oh, right, a urine catheter. I wonder why I had one this time. Not that I wasn't thankful. Seriously, when you felt like this, did you really want to be getting up and trying to sit on a low toilet? Every fifteen minutes, no less, thanks to the perpetual IV drip?

"I'm going to go get a syringe and see if we can't 'prime the pump.'" She left the room. I remembered that I'd been wearing the same tampon since quite early that morning, which creeped me out. I'd have to tell them. Christ, I couldn't reach it if my life depended on it. I told Mom. She went to tell the nurse. I lay back, staring at the ceiling and thinking, *So this is what it comes to: lying incapacitated, people drawing my urine with a syringe and changing my tampons. How demoralizing.*

Presently, they were both back, and the nurse had a huge syringe with a super sized needle on the end. I hadn't seen a syringe that big, ever. It looked like a big plastic coffee thermos. She started pulling up the blankets at my feet, looking for the little Y junction in the tube where she could insert the needle. I wondered if I would feel anything when she drew back on the plunger. She accessed the tube and drew back.

"There we go. That's more like it," she declared, satisfied, as yellow liquid filled the syringe. She'd opened the floodgates apparently because she added, "Look at that. It's really coming now. Who knew the bladder could accommodate so much?" I didn't feel a thing. I hadn't even felt like I had to pee. Funny, how that stuff works.

"OK, now we need to get that tampon outta there." She tossed the syringe out and her gloved hands pulled on the cotton cord. Out. She fixed a huge pad to me, saying that I couldn't have another tampon because the doctors were going to want to watch the blood flow carefully for clots. This simple procedure reinforced how harsh it could be staying in the hospital. No privacy. No modesty. Everything the body did was balls-to-the-wall in your face. They fed me. They bathed me. They were going to be changing my pads *and* carefully analyzing everything on them. One half of my mind took the higher road by thinking, *Well, that's medicine for you. They're professionals; they're interested in that kind of thing.* The other half was decidedly preteen: *Omigod, I can't believe other people are going to be doing that for me, it's so embarrassing!*

I slept a lot, and slept hard. If I woke up in the middle of the night or found myself alone, I amused myself by playing with my ET monitor. Time passed with a little more regularity than I remembered before. This time, three times a day, food showed up, not that I really wanted it. It was just as nasty as last time, maybe worse. Again, breakfast was the saving grace, and I'd triple up on little cereal boxes so that I could survive the rest of the meals. The surgeons had brought with them what Mom called my "Incentive Spirometer." It was a clear plastic gauge that measured air volume with a little ball and a series of blue markings like on a measuring cup. It was connected to a hose with a mouthpiece. I was supposed to inhale to raise the little ball. The first time I tried it, the ball didn't move. Not one iota. They said that before I could go home, the ball had to go up to the top line and stay there for a few seconds. It was how I could expand the remainder of my lung back to regular size.

That is how I found out that I was less almost a whole lung. When I was under the knife, when they'd opened me up and were looking for the three lobes that constitute the right lung, they could only see two, and thought that the radiation therapy may have fused two into one. Because of that, they didn't know where to cut, so they took the upper lobes, leaving the bottom third, and smallest, lobe.

I spent two days in the Peds ICU. When the time came to transfer back to 14A, they just pushed my bed right out of the room, with all my stuff on it. We went out the aquarium door and to the right. More aquariums lined the hall. Almost all the kids were sleeping, some had visitors, and everyone had the same big IV poles like I did. We went by the nurse's station where a bank of monitors—presumably one for each room—blinked and beeped, gauging what was happening inside the body of each room's resident. At the end of the hall, we went around the corner and passed the last room on the right before exiting the ICU. In it there was a small child lying in a very big bed. Every which way, tubes and wires exited her body. There were all sorts of machines and pumps and multiple IVs, all humming and pumping steadily away. It made the kid look like a big spider. I craned my neck, watching as long as I could to see if she would move, and as I rolled out of the double doors, I simultaneously gave thanks that I wasn't that child and wondered what had happened to her that would force her into such a state.

We stopped in front of the purple "C" elevators, and the transportation guy buzzed the intercom. "Be right up!" crackled a voice inside. Momentarily, the elevator door opened, and the operator smiled at us. "Come on in! Come on in! Where do you want to go today? I wouldn't mind seeing Chicago myself." I didn't say anything. I couldn't believe this guy was stuck in this elevator all day and he was *really excited* about it.

"Fourteen A" my green-jacketed transporter said. We all crammed in, he closed the doors, and we were off—up one floor. He opened the door and we rolled out.

"Have a good one!" the operator cheered.

We rolled through the double doors straight past the nurse's station and to the room at the very end of the hall. It was empty. There wasn't even a second bed. They were giving me a private room. *Sweet.* The transportation guy put my bed up against the wall facing the door, and he left. Mom pulled her big Louis Vuitton bag off the bed and tossed it on the wide windowsill. She had that look in her eyes.

"Let's rearrange your room!" she said cheerfully. Yeah. *That* look. "It'll be fun and give everyone a little more space." Some people knit or assemble puzzles for fun. Mom rearranges furniture. She gets a major charge out of it. She turned my bed to face the wall so I could see the TV on my right and out the window on my left. Then there was a ton of space on the other side nearest the door. "For visitors!" she piped.

The first few days out of a big surgery are filled with deep sleep punctuated by brief, somewhat clouded awakenings. At one point, I awoke and my hand went to my chest to press on my collarbone, a movement I had discovered to be strangely settling. Except this time it wasn't so comforting, since I felt a huge, hard, square thing sticking out of my chest. It was under the skin. I gently prodded it, suddenly wide awake. It was round and flat, like some kind of disc. What if it was some kind of freakish tumor growing there? I was very afraid.

"There's something on my chest." I said to Mom, who was sitting between the bed and the window. "There's something here, I can feel it. It might be another tumor."

She looked at me. "No, honey, that's called a porta-catheter. It's supposed to be there. They put it in while you were asleep. It's a central line. Remember last time when we saw some kids with Hickmans?" I nodded. "This is better than a Hickman, because it's totally under the skin, so you can swim and take showers without worrying about it getting wet. And just think: no more butterfly needles." Now *that* was a brilliant idea. Who decided this? Why didn't they tell me about it? I didn't understand how this thing was going to work, but just about any alternative to the Butterfly was fine with me.

Now, 14A had about forty-five beds. For those forty-five beds there was a girls' bathroom with two stalls and a shower, a boys' bathroom with the same, and a tub room with one of those big old-fashioned tubs elevated on a dais. But I wasn't mobile enough to be using these things, so every day one of my nurses would sponge bathe me. It was difficult getting used to, even though I remembered it from before. The idea of someone else washing any part of me was alien and disconcerting—what if they moved something that shouldn't move? What if they hurt me? I quickly learned there was no alternative, and I had to trust these women. The first bath was terrifying in its own right: as she moved the hot soapy cloth over my right breast, I didn't feel a thing. My entire right breast was completely numb. I didn't panic out loud, but internally my mind was racing. Did that mean it wouldn't "work" anymore? I supposed it didn't matter in the long run, but all the same, I wasn't sure I was comfortable with having a dead breast. The one saving grace was that the numbness around my other surgical site was slowly receding. Maybe the breast nerves would wake up after awhile. That thought was satisfying enough to allow for another nap.

Now that I was on 14A, every morning someone came with a portable X-ray machine to get some chest films. In order to do that, we had to finagle the thick film board behind my back against the bed. This was not a comfortable thing, clearly. First thing was to raise the head of the bed as far as it would go, almost vertical. I only had to move a few inches off the bed in order for the board to slide back there, but it was all I could to do to prop myself up with my left arm and carefully lower myself back onto the board—which was *offensively* cold, hard, and pressed oh-so-comfortably against those freakin' tubes. Then, while the technician took the next ten years to get the machine into position, I had to hold totally still.

"OK, give me one deep breath and hold it." He'd walk out of the room, press the button, the machine would emit a quick, high-pitched buzz, and it was over. Then the hard part came: propping myself back up on my left arm to get that board back out again. I'd collapse carefully back on the bed, lower the head, and nap again.

Time passed. Just like before, they tried to push Tylenol on me the day I was transferred to 14A, and just like before it was for the dogs. That Demerol machine reappeared, and again, I didn't bother using it. It didn't work anyway. Every day, at least once, they made me get up and try to walk a loop around the ward. I learned that if I bent my right arm and held it close to my side, as if in a cast, it minimized the discomfort from my surgical site. That's not really saying much, though, since the pain meds weren't working, and those tubes kept jabbing away like two screwdrivers relentlessly poking at my ribs. Every time I got up, I went from a four to a ten. My range of motion in my arm was very limited, too—I certainly couldn't raise it, so that the arm was parallel to the ground. Generally, I could make it to about quarter of the way up.

The surgeons would come in early in the morning, wake me up, and ask me how I was sleeping. The good thing about waking up then was that Dr. Rainieri was always there. He was the one with the velvety voice. Oh, *baby*. They'd ask me about my pain levels, try to get me to roll over or lean forward so they could take a peek at the incision and inspect the tubes, ask me to cough. Then they'd want to know if I'd "passed any gas." They were always asking that. I never understood what the deal was with the gas. Once, Dr. Rainieri addressed the topic of my period, and I wanted the bed to swallow me forever. *Oh, God,* I thought, *why did you have to ask* that? *Ask me anything else but that! Wake me up as early as you want, watch me vomit, whatever, but please don't ask me that.* They told me that hardcore anesthesia like this can shut down the body for a long time, and they wanted to get things moving again, so I was going to get an enema in a few days. Great. Now *there* was something to look forward to.

One day, about midmorning, Karen came in with a tray of stuff. It looked a lot like a blood draw tray, if I ever saw one, but there was no butterfly.

"What's that?" I asked.

"This," she said, setting the tray down, "is for accessing your port. We're gonna get rid of those nasty IVs and replace them with this." I looked on the tray. There were iodine packets, alcohol swabs, sterile gloves, big clear plastic stickers called op sites, plenty of tape, cotton balls, and a plastic packet inside of which a tube was coiled. It had clamps on it and Y-junctions; the tube came from the end of a thick needle that was bent at a right angle. She pulled the neck of my gown down to reveal the flat circular protrusion from my chest.

"Did they tell you about it?" she asked.

I said, "Yeah, a little. They said what it was, but not how it worked." Karen had me feel it and described how it worked. A plastic disc, it has a rubber center out of which a tube runs, and is anchored into the body. The whole thing is stitched into place and the tube goes straight into one of my major veins.

"Then, we take this," she pointed to the bent needle and tubes, "and we plug into the rubber part. It's bent, right, so it lays flat against your chest once it's in there. We tape it down, cover it with an op site, and away you go." She started to work. She opened the iodine pouch and swabbed the whole area, and then cleaned it with a few alcohol swabs. Then, she got rid of the first pair of gloves and carefully slipped on the sterile ones. She opened the needle package and felt for the rubber part of the port under my skin; then she pressed the needle through and into the disc.

"Ow!" I yelped, flinching. It was a very uncomfortable feeling, having a needle, a fairly large one as needles go, poked through at the chest.

"Good, good. Good return, good flow," she said. She had a saline-filled syringe and was pushing it through the line. It was cold, and I could feel the coldness in my chest. She stopped pushing and pulled back on the plunger; blood rushed into the syringe, mixing with the water. "Good return," she nodded approvingly. She pushed the rest of the syringe through, placed a cotton ball underneath the "wings" of the bent needle, and taped it down securely. Over all of it, she placed the large, plastic op site. She hooked it up to the IV line and restarted the flow.

"Good stuff, huh?" she asked. "Sure beats those old IVs on your wrists." She proceeded to remove the tape on my IVs and pull them out. They were sore, and they left little scars that are still visible today. I liked this port thing. It was totally under my shirt, and I had free range of motion with my wrists—I always did, really, but having an IV in the back of my hand or alongside my radius near the wrist joint always made me feel like I didn't.

Since the Tylenol wasn't working and I didn't even bother with the Demerol, telling the doctors and nurses that it was pointless (they always argued, "But you can take it every ten minutes!"), at some point they switched me to a new pain med. I don't know what it was, but it was intense. One night, somehow, I was given too much, and though still conscious, I started hallucinating and babbling incoherently. As my parents were getting ready to leave for the night, I begged them to take the chickens off my hands because they were scratching me. And they were! A fat white hen and a mottled black-and-white hen were perched on the backs of my hands, scratching away. They were drawing blood. Mom tried to tell me that there were no chickens on my hands. After they left, Denise, my preferred swing-shift nurse, came in and saw that

I wasn't breathing very much. By this time, the hens had left and I was just in a dazed state of half-sleep, wanting only to drift off. My eyelids were made of iron. She pressed hard on my hand.

"Lindsey, I need you to wake up." I opened my eyes and looked at her dopily, then closed them again. She pressed the call button and the intercom buzzed. "We need to order an oxygen tank. Now." Someone crackled on the other end. I heard her pull up Mom's chair on the left side, and she sat there, poking my arm every few seconds, keeping me awake.

The pump droned.

I wanted to sleep.

Poke.

"Lindsey, wake up. I need you to take a big breath for me."

I took as big of a breath as I dared, not very big.

"Lindsey, I need you to take another one. Breathe for me. Breathe big."

I breathed.

The tiny motor in the IV pump whirred as it pushed fluid into my body. Sleep...

"Lindsey, wake up!" Poke. "Breathe!" I opened my eyes, turned my head, and looked at her. I blinked hard, struggling to keep them open. I *wanted* to do what she said, but I *couldn't*. "I'm staying with you until the oxygen gets here," she said loudly, "because you're not breathing enough. Again. Breathe." Dang it! Why couldn't I sleep? I tried to tell her all I was going to do was take a little nap, but the only thing that came out was slurred noise.

Poke.

I breathed.

After what felt like an eternity, someone else came into the room, and Denise jumped up. She fixed something under my nose that went into my nostrils. I heard her rustling around on my right, and air suddenly blew out of the tube into my nose. Then I was awake—well, more awake. What was *this* thing? How could I sleep with this air blowing into my head? I tried to push it away. She put it back.

"OK, now you can sleep. Just breathe normally, and you'll be fine." She fussed over something else before leaving. I drunkenly watched her leave, and then turned to face the wall in front of me again. I was tired, but this air thing was pretty obnoxious. I wasn't sure I'd actually be able to get to sleep.

The next morning I woke up with the surgeons looking expectantly at me. The air-blowing tube was gone. Had I dreamed all that?

"Are you sleeping well?" Dr. Rainieri asked, flashing his perfect smile. *Oh, Armando, who cares if I slept well, everything is just fine now that you're here.* We went through the average exercises: have a look at the site, the tubes, try to cough, etc.

Walking had become slightly easier, but I was still in that phase where one false move could bring me to my knees, and then I'd really be in a pickle. In pain and on the floor with no easy way to get up. So, walking still took two helpers, one on either side. One person would be in charge of the IV pole and provide secondary arm support; the other person would be the primary arm support. Slowly, slowly, we made our way around the ward. The first time I made a full circle was a day for celebration, so I climbed back in bed and slept. One day I had been for a walk with just Mom, and when I was sitting back on the bed and starting to lean back toward the mattress, all my back muscles seized up. I couldn't move, and moreover, I was afraid to even try, thinking that forcing it would cause worse pain. I wouldn't let Mom help me—I didn't trust her to not unwittingly hurt me. She dashed from the room yelling for help while I remained in that awkward, despairingly uncomfortable (to say the least) position until a couple nurses came running back, supported me by the shoulders and sides, and lowered me into bed, not without discomfort. When I hit the pillow, I didn't even care that the tubes had resumed their annoying jabbing sensations; it was a full-body relief to be lying down again.

Days passed. Dr. Wolff would come in, wash up, and examine me. The surgeons would do the same. Denise pulled my urine catheter, and I was forced to get up to pee all the time—and I mean *all* the time; all those liters of water go in and they have to come back out. The pain was never controlled. I was never comfortable. More importantly, I am a born stomach-sleeper, and I couldn't even roll myself onto my stomach without hurting myself. So, after the anesthesia wore off, I was having difficulty sleeping.

The best we could do was get a few nurses to prop a line of pillows to one side and slowly push me onto my side, partly lying on the pillows. It was enough to encourage a couple hours' sleep. Then I would wake up, get help rolling back onto my back, and sleep again. It was a day of triumph when I was able to roll myself on and off the pillows.

On the 3rd night out of surgery, one of the surgical residents came by. I wondered where the rest of his pack was, as though he were a lone wolf, and simultaneously lamented that he wasn't Dr. Rainieri.

"OK, Lindsey. It's the big day. Those tubes are coming out. Your pneumothorax has been getting smaller and now it's gone, so we don't need those things anymore."

Good. I couldn't wait to get rid of them. I flattened my bed, and he and the nurse helped roll me onto my stomach.

"OK, two things: first, I need you to relax all the way. I'm going to count to three, and on three you need to breathe in, hold your breath, and I'll pull. *Do not breathe until I say so.*"

"Why?" I asked.

"Because if you breathe while I'm trying to take them out, we'll have to put them back in."

"Yeah, but you'll put me to sleep for that, right?"

"No, we'd have to do it immediately, right now."

I froze. He wanted me to *relax* after that? Crazy man.

He continued, "After they're out, you're going to feel two tiny bee stings while I tie the threads that we put in there ahead of time. I have to close the little holes." *Bee stings, schmee stings.* All I cared about was not screwing up this breathing thing.

"Are you ready?" he asked as he slowly peeled the tape off.

"No!" I squeaked, terrified and on the verge of tears.

"Lindsey, we have to do this," he said, very softly, "When these are out, I promise you you'll sleep like a baby. You'll feel a lot better." I thought for a second. There was no choice. They *had* to come out sometime, and they sure were a pain in the...chest. Just get it done and over with. I sighed inwardly. "OK. Go." I could feel the flat of his gloved hand pressing down on my back, bracing himself.

"One..." I closed my eyes, on the verge of tears. *Don't cry, you don't want to breathe...*

"Two…" Tears swelled between my eyelids, Here it comes…

"Three!" I inhaled and held it. Just as I did, I felt something being ripped in seeming slow motion from inside my chest as I heard a low tearing noise emanate from within. I felt the ends of the tubes dragging through my body under the ribs, like tires leaving hot skid marks on pavement. *Oh, God, this can't be real. This is a nightmare,* I thought. I almost screamed but caught it in my throat at the last second, remembering what he'd said about not breathing.

Then they popped out.

Though I could still feel the burning, aching sensation where they had just been, as though they had scratched me hard from the inside, the comparative relief was immense and instantaneous. I heard him throw the tubes in the trash. Then, I felt his fingers again on my back. *Zing!* He tied the first knot—that skin around the entry hole for the tubes is so sensitive. *Zing!* He tied the second. And he was right. It did feel like a giant bee sting. I heard him snip the ends of the threads before he said, "OK, Lindsey, let's roll you back onto your back." They helped shove me back over, and I was stunned with disbelief that it was almost painless. He stood there talking to me, but I wasn't listening. I was looking past him into the trash where the tubes stuck out the top. They looked enormous. I couldn't believe that I lived with those things in my chest for almost four days. I was suddenly exhausted.

He left the room, and my mother followed him, still conversing. I could hear bits of what they were saying, but I stared fixedly at the tubes, covered in blood and mucous, dripping a little now and then. Mom's voice broke in and out in the hallway. "…control her pain…can't function…not working…" I could tell from the tone that she was giving him a talking to. And she should. The pain had been ridiculously unbearable. I think if she'd known his middle name, she would have used it for effect like she'd done with me so many times. I could hear it in my mind: *Lindsey MICHELLE! You get back here and…* You can fill in the rest. Coming back to the present, I heard Dr. Bellos mumble something indistinguishable in response.

"Thank you. That will be great," Mom said as she opened the door and came back in my room. Partway through, she turned around to him again and said, "We'll see you kids tomorrow morning, right?" Then her face turned red and she froze like a deer in headlights, eyes wide. "I mean," she stammered, "it's just that, all of you are so much younger than me...so it's like you're kids...you know..." she finished lamely. I laughed silently at the whole scenario. The resident had this bland smile on his face and nodded, excusing himself. Mom turned to me, the red starting to fade in her face and neck. She walked up to the side of my bed.

"Good news, Booie," she cheerfully exclaimed. "They're going to give you a new pain med. It's like the Cadillac of pain control. He says it's like taking a giant Advil. It won't make you feel weird like the narcotics. And guess what? He thinks you might be the first kid to ever have it. Cool, huh?"

Hmm. I looked back at her and wondered, *If this medicine is so great, why haven't they tried it before?*

She continued, "The only thing is that the first dose has to be an injection in your muscle, but after that they can put it in the IV."

Ah, there's the catch. A muscle injection? You've got to be kidding. I frowned. I knew what those needles looked like. I used the same kind to give the horse her shots. I didn't want one of those anywhere near me. *But then again...if it'll actually work...*

Denise came in with the dose. The needle was huge compared to the butterfly I was so loathingly accustomed to. I lifted the head of my bed so I could sit up, still adjusting to the stunning ease of it all after the chest tubes had been removed. Denise lifted the blanket at my right thigh and swiped the skin with an alcohol pad. She uncapped the needle, looking at me, at the ready. "How do you want to do this? Should I count to three? You want to tell me when to go?" I planted my hands down on the bed on either side of my quad and stared at the needle, thinking. She suggested, "Maybe you should turn your head? Look at your mom?"

I concentrated on my leg. "Count to three, then just go," I decided. When the needle thrust into my muscle, my hands clenched and flew up around the syringe as if I thought I'd grab it from her and do it myself. But I held back. She pushed the meds in a flash and I fell back on the bed, totally drained.

It worked almost instantly.

It *was* like an enormous Advil. I wasn't groggy or spacey, and I could move without much restriction. I still couldn't raise that right arm up higher than my shoulder, but things were good. The next day I felt like I could sprint around the ward with just one helper, and was able to keep walking for as many as five laps at a time. That afternoon, lunch appeared (I smelled it long before it actually came through the door). When Karen lifted the lid on the plate, there were three pieces of fried chicken, some mashed potatoes, and carrot sticks accompanied by cranberry juice and finished with a square of chocolate cake. I felt like I'd never been so hungry in my life. I easily got out of bed and sat up in the chair that Mom slept in. Mom pushed my bed table over to me with the tray on it. I sat there and gulped fried chicken just like it was any old lunch on any old day.

As I was finishing my cake, Dr. Bellos returned to check in. Mom started gushing about the new drug—Toradol they called it—and how great it was (and it *is*), and how much I'd walked, and how easily I could move. Dr. Bellos asked if I would cough for him. I swallowed a mouthful of cake—*man*, did it taste good—paused for a second, and produced a hearty cough. No pain. I was surprised. He seemed satisfied, requested a urine sample, announced they'd be back later in the afternoon or early evening, and left.

He returned later that day—where was Dr. Rainieri?—and did an exam. He took each of my hands and asked me to pull against his resistance. No problem. He had me cough, then take a hard long pull on the incentive spirometer. I got the little ball to the top and rattled it around up there before running out of air and letting it drop. He asked me how many laps I'd done that day.

"Five or six," I answered.

"Good that's great." He started ticking points off on his fingers. "Your pneumothorax is gone, you've been detached, you're walking, your appetite's back, and you're doing well on the spirometer. I think you can go home tomorrow."

"That's fantastic!" Mom exclaimed.

"We'll all be by at one point or another tomorrow to do one last check and fill out the discharge papers." He looked at us both. "Good job," he said, smiling gently.

After he left, Mom immediately started bustling about, packing stuff up. Linda has never been one to wait patiently around. She likes to take charge.

Karen came in later and said we had to go to the playroom because she was going to teach me something. So, I grabbed a hold of my "Pole-ish" friend and followed her to the playroom across the hall from my room. Mom followed. On a table in there were a few oranges, a plush doll, alcohol swabs, some tiny syringes, little needles, and little vials of saline. One of my friends at school had diabetes, and these needles and little containers looked exactly like the ones she used. Karen sat us down. "We're learning to do subcutaneous injections," she announced. "That means 'under the skin.'"

"Why do I need to know that?" I asked, dumbly.

"Because Dr. Wolff wants you to give yourself a hormone shot called G-CSF after you're done with every chemo cycle. It'll help your white count bounce back a lot faster."

"*What?*" I was incredulous. Oh, very nice. When we started talking about surgery and stuff, nobody mentioned getting—no wait, *giving* myself—shots at home. What was this? "I have to give myself shots? Why can't you just put it through my port?"

"G-CSF is a different kind of drug. It doesn't come in pills, and it doesn't work very well intravenously, so we can't put it through your port. It really works well when you inject it just under your skin and your body can absorb it."

"So, it doesn't go in a vein at all?" I asked, tilting my head up but maintaining eye contact with her. She held up both her hands. "Nope."

I looked over at Mom, who tried to be positive. "It won't be that hard, Booie," she reassured me. "You'll just stick it in, shoot it, and you're out. It'll be really fast and easy." Well, obviously it would be for *Linda*, bless her heart. Karen showed us how to do everything correctly: clean the site with alcohol swabs, and don't blow on it to dry it (which is tantamount to pouring a beaker of bacteria on it). Then, she showed us how to screw the needle into the syringe, uncap the needle, wipe off the vial with an alcohol pad, and draw the fluid out of it. She instructed me on tapping the syringe to get the bubbles out and then told me where I could take the shot.

"There are three places that will be good. Your upper arm, your stomach, and your thigh. The important thing is to do it where you have some good fat under the skin. The stomach is the least sensitive." I remembered that from my friend Jennifer who had diabetes. She told us all that she put the insulin shots in her stomach because it hurt less. None of us, I think, believed her. I thought for a second that it might be a good idea, since I still had so many numb spots from my kidney surgery. But the idea of plunging a needle—no matter how small—into my stomach was too unnerving. I practiced on the orange, and so did Mom. The orange squirted Mom in the eye.

"You think you got it?" Karen asked me.

"Yeah, I got it. It's not that hard."

"So no problem? You can do this?"

I looked at her sideways. "I don't have much of a choice. Dr. Wolff is the Big Dog. What he says, goes." I sighed heavily. At least I didn't have to start doing this right away. No one had even brought up the topic of when chemo would start. I was just thankful they hadn't gotten it underway during my surgical recovery, like last time.

I spent the rest of the day in my room, mellowing out, thinking about what had just happened and what I would be expected to do in the next six months. When the light outside started to get longer and more orange, Mom said, "I'm going home soon, and then I'll bring you back some clothes to wear home tomorrow." She was happy as a clam.

When I was on my own that night, even though my pain was a one on a scale of ten, I still felt exhausted. I fell asleep easily, and finally, I rejoiced in being able to roll myself over onto my stomach and side without any pain or problems. Small victories.

The next morning, Dr. Wolff and his entourage came by. He went through the usual motions: wash up in the foot-pedal-activated sink, dry hands on paper towels, take a listen, take a peek, tell me I should come back to the clinic in a week to discuss when we'd start chemo again, or even *if* we'd start chemo again.

"If?" I asked, surprised. I'd assumed that's what happened any time you have cancer removed. Besides, they'd just bothered to teach me that whole shot thing.

He leaned his head a little to one side and kind of pushed his shoulders up into an almost-shrug. "There is some debate as to whether it's truly necessary. The margins of your tumor were negative for 'feelers,' and there are no other detectable signs of Wilms anywhere else in your body. But we'll talk about that next week. I'll have Kaylee call you for an appointment." I watched him walk out, hands in the pockets of his impossibly short coat. *Huh,* I thought. *Maybe this won't be so bad after all. Maybe I'm done.*

Later on in the day, after Mom had arrived, the surgical herd arrived. Finally, the whole group was there: Dr. Henricks—who'd done the first operation on me—Dr. Rainieri—who was just pretty as pretty can be—and of course, Dr. Bellos who bore an incredible resemblance to a young Anthony Edwards. We went through the motions again: spirometer, look at the site, listen, check out the films, strength testing, coughing. They were all very pleased. They said someone would be back with the discharge orders later, and that I would need to get the stitches at the tube site pulled in two weeks.

"We don't want you getting things wet, yet, and any time your port is accessed, be careful not to let the water get under the op site; we don't want any infections."

After they left, Mom continued to get ready to leave. "I want you to go take a shower before we go home," she said to me.

"But Dr. Henricks said not to get anything wet." I argued.

She got the Mom Look on her face. "You'll be fine. Dry off really well."

I tried to argue with her, but what Mama Linda says, goes. Karen unhooked me from my IV, and I went off to take a shower. It felt so good to have hot water running over skin that had been pressed into a mattress for the better part of a week. When I came out and walked back to the room, I was wearing a pair of elastic pants and a white T-shirt covered in drawings of horses and riders. I came around the corner and saw my room. Outside of it were Dr. Bellos, Mom, and the red wagon full of our stuff. He looked at me.

"There's one thing, though, that we need to talk about. Your urine sample showed trace amounts of hemoglobin in it." I froze, thinking of my kidney, my heart racing. I stared at Mom, and started to say something, but he continued, "...but you're still on your period, correct?" He looked at me. I nodded, relieved instantly. "Then that is almost undoubtedly what it is. I wouldn't think anymore about it."

Stupid period, always ruined everything. At least my *heart* was working fine.

At home that night, I faced a peculiar, but not unfamiliar, set of dilemmas: first, there would be no nurse to automatically update my Toradol overnight, and second, the bed didn't move up and down, so this would be my first experience with trying to sit up and lie down without depending on the incline of the mattress. I felt anxious. With Mom's help, I was able to lower myself to the mattress and roll over, but lying flat on my stomach caused pressure in the small of my back. "Bring your right leg up a little," Mom suggested. I bent my leg slightly and it worked. I was asleep instantly.

The next morning, I woke up pretty sore but tolerable. Now I felt like I could get away with Tylenol, so I took a couple and went into the living room. Mom came in from outside where she'd been weeding her flower beds. "It's really beautiful outside, Booie, you should come out and sit for a while." I thought for a little while and declined. "Come on," she insisted. "It will be good for you to have a little sun. Come on. Time to make some vitamin D." She brought one of the kitchen chairs outside and set it in the grass near where she was working. Holding my right arm bent against my side, I lowered myself into the chair using my left arm. The sun didn't feel good, it felt *great*. I gotta hand it to Mom. She's right a lot. I took in the homey sights and smells: the maples bordering the riverbanks were just starting to turn; the wheat stubble made the fields look like soft, dull gold; and the smell of fresh dirt from the flower beds was a little piece of heaven. Sassy and Sandy Dunes lay down around my chair, panting in the morning sunlight. The goat bleated at us, watching with his ears pricked, wanting off his chain to be a part of the herd. I sat there and listened to Mom weed and talk about going back to school, my upcoming birthday, and the miscellany of things that I'd missed in the last week.

Kaylee

Kids are so resilient because they don't internalize anything. They think, this sucks and then they go play. They'll be eating pizza, then they'll puke, and then they want to know where the rest of their pizza is. I love that resiliency. That's just how they are, and they aren't over thinking anything.

Sitting on the butcher paper spread out over the hard-cushioned exam table, I stared at a colorful print on the wall of a psychedelic cartoon cow with enormous hooves and nose, chewing on a stalk of grass. On the wall behind me was a poster emblazoned with "Everything I Need to Know About Life I Learned From My Cat." Below the title was a picture of a fat tabby, an impish look in its eyes. Below the cat were printed lines like, "When in doubt, cop an attitude," or "Laps are most inviting when the sewing is already there," and "The only respectable place for a nap is on top of the clean laundry."

Dr. Wolff appeared in the doorway, hands in his coat pockets with his default half-smile gracing his face. He asked us how things were while he washed and dried his thin hands, and chatted comfortably for a while before tossing the paper towel and reaching up just underneath my jaw to prod my lymph nodes. His hands smelled like the antibacterial soap they use. They always smelled like that. It's a sterile, acrid smell that permeates every room, hallway, gown, and blanket in the hospital. I remained silent while he looked me over, and he continued chatting easily with Mom before pulling out the stethoscope and rubbing the bell furiously on the palm of his hand in a vain attempt to warm it. He poked the bell down the collar of my shirt onto my sternum saying, "It's still a little cold." I inhaled sharply; ooh, boy, it *was* cold. *If I were a doctor*, I thought, *I'd keep a hot pack in my pocket and stick the bell in there.* After he was done, he asked me to hop down and pull up my shirt in the back, where he looked briefly at the thin red line before listening to my lungs.

When he was done, he crossed his thin arms, stuffing the stethoscope back in its default pocket. He looked at me. "Let's talk about what we're going to do next."

"OK," Mom said, leaning forward. I watched him. He continued, nodding to Mom. "We talked briefly about the idea of maybe not doing chemo?" Mom and I both murmured assent. "OK." He had a template for deep thought, and that was looking up, mouth slightly open, punctuating his thoughts with lingering sounds. "Ahhh…Dr. Stein, Dr. Norman, and I think it would be a good idea to go ahead with it. Being that you had a late-stage tumor, it'd be good to make sure everything is cleaned up in there." I experienced a split second of disappointment, but I knew deep down that he was right.

"So when do you want to start?" he asked me.

"When do *I* want to start? I don't have to start today?" I asked, stunned that it was my decision.

"No," he replied, not breaking eye contact.

I thought for a minute or so before responding. "Let's start after my birthday, then," I announced.

"October thirteenth, right?" he confirmed. He nodded repeatedly, mumbling "OK…mmhmm…OK" to himself while he thought. "Let me get a calendar," he said as he walked out of the room and down the hall. He returned with the scheduler in his hands, turning the pages to October. "The thirteenth is a Wednesday. Why don't we see you in here on Thursday the fourteenth?"

I shrugged.

"Kaylee will access your port, and we'll do the infusion. It's going to be a five-day cycle, so on the weekend you'll have to go to Fourteen A—"

I cut him off. "Huh-uh. I don't want to do this as an outpatient. I hated that. I want to have them all in the hospital."

He looked at me hard. "Oh, now, come on," he said, as if what I said was the most ridiculous thing he'd ever heard, "there's no reason you can't do this as an outpatient. It's good for you to be at home."

I threw up my hands and looked at him wide-eyed. "What's wrong with the hospital? It's the cleanest place I could be—"

This time *he* interrupted *me*, scoffing, "Hospitals are filthy! Just about the dirtiest place you could be. It's much cleaner–and safer– at your house."

I considered this and wondered how it could be true when there were staff wandering through cleaning that place day and night. "I just don't want to be at home and have to take everything by mouth and stuff. I feel better when I can put everything in the IV." Also, I wanted a very controlled environment. I wasn't going to go through the hell of it like before. Having a nurse, a doctor on call, an adjustable bed, and cable TV all *right there* were very comforting ideas. So, after a short argument, I won. He'd admit me for every cycle of chemo.

Just then, Mom piped up. "Dr. Wolff, I wanted to ask you about pets. Is it OK to have the pets around her all the time?"

"Generally," he nodded. "What kinds of pets do you have?"

"We have a couple dogs and a few cats and a bird."

"Dogs are definitely fine. Cats are actually dirtier than dogs…"

"Really?" we both asked in unison, surprised. I wondered how an animal could bathe constantly and be dirtier than a dog. That's what you get when you lick yourself, I guess.

"…but they are generally fine, too. I would recommend giv- ing the bird away. Birds are especially dirty and carry a lot of bac- teria." So, Travis's blue parakeet, Doodles, which we'd only had for a couple months, was outta there. Wolff continued, "The dogs are especially good if you have a small one. One that can sit with her in bed. Pet therapy is fantastic." Occasionally they had pet therapy dogs come through the wards. Often they were big black Newfoundlands that pulled kids around in a wagon. I preferred Sandy Dunes.

There was no need for blood that day, so we left with an appoint- ment on the books for Thursday October 14. Before we left, Dr. Wolff gave us a stack of information on what drugs I would be taking and how they worked. He looked at me, thick eyebrows raised, and said, "Read up on that. I'm going to give you a test."

"What?" I asked incredulously. "Oh, yeah, right."

"No, seriously! Be ready for a test." The pitch of his voice would always raise a couple notches and his eyebrows would travel skyward, wrinkling his forehead if he were being serious or excited about something. That's when you knew he meant it, and that scared me. I had to memorize this stuff. I couldn't disappoint him. What if his test was really hard? After all, he was a *professor of medicine*. I wondered what kinds of tests he gave his medical students, and how many of the students I had seen were his students. Did anyone ever flunk his class? Dr. Neidermeyer, who'd diagnosed me in the ER and sent me to Doernbecher, had once been a student of Dr. Wolff's. I was going to study my butt off.

"Oh, I almost forgot!" Mom exclaimed, stopping and turning back to the desk. "How do you think we should tell all the kids and parents at Lindsey's school? Is there anything in particular they should know this time, I mean, aside from the whole chicken pox thing like before?"

He looked pensive for a moment. "It may be a good idea for me and either Kaylee, or Patsy to actually come out and talk to the class. They probably have questions about what's happening and what happened before. Let me see if we can schedule that. Why don't you contact her school and see if they would be willing?"

Huh, so Dr. Wolff was going to come out to my school. Sweet. I was proud that I'd get to show him off to my friends and they'd see how smart and cool he was.

My first day back at school, Mom and I talked to my teacher and the principal about Dr. Wolff coming out for a lecture on my disease. They thought it would be a good idea and were going to look into scheduling it. There had also been rumors about the eighth graders taking a trip to Washington, DC, right after graduation; and we would all start fundraising in the next few weeks by picking apples, having car washes, bake sales, etc. My heart sank, realizing that with treatment, the reality of my going out to wash cars and pick apples was very slim, not to mention the idea of being around food and smelling baked goods at a sale. Looked like I wouldn't be going to Washington, DC.

The school ended up scheduling Dr. Wolff to come out to speak to my class for an hour during the following week. The night before they were to visit, we happened to be out to dinner with Sharon, and her husband, Dr. John Dogan–the oncologist at the hospital where I was first diagnosed in the ER. We were at a Mexican restaurant in Hillsboro, my favorite place for giant burritos. As we sat under the paper-mache parrots crunching on chips and salsa, we discussed my newest disease. Mom asked Dr. Dogan all sorts of questions, some of which he couldn't answer, as he explained that pediatric cancers are very different from adult cancers. Periodically he asked me some questions.

"Will you be taking Neupogen?"

"Neupogen. What's that?" I asked.

"It's a hormone that helps stimulate your white cells."

"Oh, yeah, they called it G-CSF."

"Yeah, mm-hm," he said, crunching away, "they call it that, too."

"What's it called again? The real name?" I asked.

"Neupogen. Filgrastim Neupogen."

Neupogen, huh? That was a lot easier to say than G-CSF, where I always thought I was mixing up letters.

"What about Zofran? Have they mentioned that yet?" he asked, reaching for more chips.

"No," I said warily, imagining some new fantastically monstrous pill or serum that tasted as bad as the liquid sulfamethoxazole. "What's Zofran?" Now here was a name I wouldn't forget—it's not like the letter Z gets used that often, anyway, but in a drug it really stood out.

He nodded at me. "Mhm. Good stuff. They'll give it to you an hour before you get your chemo and you won't get sick."

I was stunned. "*What?*" Now this was getting exciting. It all sounded too good to be true. Could they actually prevent you from getting sick? When? How? I needed to be a part of this.

"Yeah, we've been using it for a while. If they don't automatically give it to you, you should ask about it. Sometimes pediatrics don't have the same stuff available as the adults do. But it should work the same on you as it would on a grown-up."

I don't think I really believed him, or at least I thought it would be one of those drugs I wouldn't be able to get. Eventually, someone brought up that Dr. Wolff would be visiting my class so that we could ask questions. John thought that was a good idea. He turned back to me. "What are *you* going to ask him?"

"Me? I don't know." I thought for a second. I wanted to make sure I asked a good one. Dr. Wolff was pretty danged smart so I wanted him to think I was a smart kid. "Hey, will you help me come up with a good question for him?"

John looked toward the ceiling, thinking for a second. "OK." He tore a scrap of paper from a little pocket notebook and started writing on it. "Here's a good one," he continued. "How about 'If I get anemia, can I have erythropoietin?'" He handed the paper to me. I examined his chicken-scratch question, trying to decipher it.

"I don't know if I can even say that. Erthro...poten?" I said lamely.

"No, no. *Erythropoietin.*" He emphasized the syllables. I took his pen and spelled the name of the drug out phonetically, like they do in the dictionary.

"Ee...rith...row...poe...eat...in," I finished. "What is that, anyway?"

He was chewing away again on the chips. "It's a lot like the Neupogen. Although it doesn't work nearly as well. But in theory it's supposed to help you make more red cells so you won't be so tired and you can avoid transfusions." He shrugged. "In theory."

This is a good question, I thought. This'll totally get him.

Oh yeah, right.

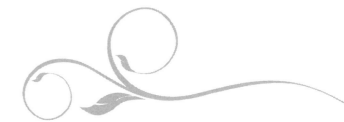

The next day at school, Dr. Wolff was supposed to show up right after our break. When we were released from class for fifteen minutes, I stayed at the big wooden double doors that faced the parking strip along the road, looking through the little panes for the Wolff-man. About halfway through the break, a boxy bright orange Volvo turned onto Visitation Road, slowed, and turned into the parking strip. I saw a thin man and a woman with short curly hair—unmistakably Dr. Wolff and another one of my nurses, Nancy—step out of the car. She stooped in to get some things out of the back seat, one of which looked like a big plastic torso. It had boobs. I wondered if the boys in my class would laugh at it. The bell rang, and everyone came rushing back to the classroom from break.

I was nervous. No one else was, and they milled around talking. I sat in my desk quietly, waiting. Our teacher, a fat man with glasses and a dark beard, walked in. Everyone clammed up immediately and sat down. He announced that we were skipping English that day for a guest speaker. "Lindsey's doctor is here to explain to you what is going on, and you will be free to ask him questions about cancers or treatments or anything. It will be an open forum. *Do not* be disrespectful. These people have driven a long way to talk to us today."

Everyone was suddenly very expectant. Some looked at me, some whispered to each other, some looked at Holly who they knew to be closely in cahoots with me. A few minutes later, the principal escorted Dr. Wolff and Nancy to the classroom. He looked weird to me. I'd never seen him without his white coat, and today he was wearing a regular sport coat. He also had glasses on. Where did those things come from? I found this somehow disconcerting, but I kept my mouth shut.

"Why are you wearing glasses?" Holly brazenly shouted out. Oh, good, at least *someone* asked.

"Because the State of Oregon says I have to, if I want to drive a motor vehicle," he responded, smiling his characteristic half-smile. Nancy set the plastic, breasted torso on the desk and a small box next to it. Dr. Wolff introduced himself and her and started to talk about what cancer was.

It can be hard to describe the science of cancer to anyone, let alone children, but it had been a part of my life for so long it was easy for me to absorb. I learned a few things about the disease that I hadn't known before—like the oldest woman to ever be diagnosed with Wilms was in her thirties. At one point, Nancy picked up the torso, which had a flap on it above one of the breasts and started to describe my porta-catheter: where it was installed, how it worked, what it did, why it was helpful, how it was better than a Hickman line, which is like an IV permanently anchored into your chest that feeds into your main vessels. She opened the little box and pulled one out so everyone could see the flat plastic disc with the rubber center and the long flexible plastic tube. It looked like a giant flat sperm.

When Dr. Wolff opened up the floor to questions, at first, nobody moved. So I raised my hand and asked my smart aleck question. "If I get anemia, can I have erythropoietin?" I barely was able to enunciate the word properly. He frowned a little, deep in thought, described what anemia is to the class, and proceeded to answer my question. For a second I thought I'd got him. Then he started in on the answer, describing what erythropoietin was and how it was supposed to work. But I didn't even listen to his answer; I was impressed that he could pull this information straight off the top of his head—just like he always could do with the tiniest facts from my history and presumably every other one of his patients' histories. I wondered if he ever looked things up in textbooks, if he ever failed to come up with an answer. I came out of my reverie when one of my classmates asked a question.

"You said that chicken pox can kill her even though she's already had it?"

"That's right," said Dr. Wolff, hands in his coat pockets.

"So...if all of her antibodies are affected, then will she have to get all of her vaccinations again? I mean, later when she finishes chemo?"

Dr. Wolff looked pensive and surprised at the same time. "You mean things like Tetanus or Measles, not the flu shot, right?" he clarified. The boy nodded. Dr. Wolff cocked his head a bit to one side and looked up as is his wont when thinking, "Excellent question, and I'm not sure there is an answer to it, officially. In our experience, we've never had problems with patients recovering and then contracting the diseases that they were immunized against as infants. So in all likelihood, no, she won't." He nodded. "Next question?"

They asked about everything: why does the hair fall out, why do patients get sick, how do the drugs work, and so forth. When everyone had finished asking, our teacher concluded the session, and Dr. Wolff and Nancy left, taking the bare-breasted torso with them.

I continued to go to school like normal for the next few weeks. A few days before my birthday, on a Saturday evening, Holly called and asked me if I wanted to come over. I asked Mom and she said yes but that we'd better go now because she had somewhere to be that night. I was wearing a pair of stretch pants, a T-shirt with horses on it, and a grungy pair of Keds. I'd just returned from the horse barn so things were a little dusty, but not dirty. Mom examined me up and down and said disparagingly, "Don't you want to change your clothes before we go?"

I gave her a weird look. "Why?" I snorted. "I'm just going to Holly's house."

She looked me in the eye and said, "I really think you should change."

I became recalcitrant. "Why should I have to change? She won't care. Why do you all of a sudden?" I grabbed an overnight bag and headed out the door as Mom threw up her hands in exasperation. I didn't notice how well dressed she was because she was always well dressed and made up before going out in public. The woman won't even walk into a grocery store without a quick coat of lipstick.

When we got to Holly's house—a big gray and white Victorian with maroon trim built in the late twenties—I got out of the car and headed for the back door. Mom stopped me and shouted, "I think you should go in the front door!"

Now this was getting weird. I scoffed at her. "*Mom*! I never go through the front door." Something was up. "Why are you coming in anyway?"

She looked at me, almost taken aback for a moment. But she recovered quickly. "Because. *I'm the Mom*!" she boomed. Whatever. So I went in through the back door into the kitchen and Holly and her mom were sitting in there around the island. I put my stuff down by the door, and Holly said, "Hey, come in here. You gotta check this out." She was walking toward the door to the dining room. We walked in, and she turned on the light. The room was full of people: classmates, former classmates, cousins, friends, Aunt Jeanna. They all yelled, "*Surprise!*"

Aha! So this was it! They were throwing me a *surprise* party! Everything made sense instantly. Happy birthday to *me*!

We had good times that night. There was Mexican food—my favorite— and Mom made us play a game called "Toilet Paper Bride" where we paired up and one person had to use a roll of TP to dress the other in a wedding gown in two minutes. Even Holly's dad got into the game—he was a bride, and all us thirteen-year-old girls thought it hilarious that a guy was going to wear a toilet paper dress. Mostly, though, we all just did what thirteen-year-old girls do: hang out.

At the end of the party after most people had gone home, a woman came to the door. She had a mastiff puppy in her arms.

"Ohhh, who's the little bay-bee?" Mom cooed while she scratched its head.

"This is Lindsey's present!" my friend Julie exclaimed, smiling.

"What?" Mom and I exclaimed together. I thought it was great. Mom did not. The puppy was a she, and she was very *heavy*. At only three months old, she weighed almost thirty pounds. She was very shy, and when we put her on the couch next to Mom, she buried her head between Mom and the couch. Mom looked skeptical at first, but then loosened up right away. "Oh, hello, baby, don't be scared...don't be scared." She picked her up. "Hi there, baby. Oh, look at *you*, aren't you a big girl?" She held up the puppy and said, "Hey, we finally have a dog that is as big-boned as I am!"

Julie's mom had brought the dog. She handed us an envelope, saying, "She's a purebred, so here are her papers. You can register her name when you pick one out."

Long after everyone else had left, we were still there with our new puppy. Mom said, "I never thought I'd say this, but it's a good thing your Dad is in the ICU right now. He would *freak out* if he knew someone gave you a dog for your birthday."

"What, didn't they ask you first?" I asked.

"Nope! What should we name her?" Everyone started shooting off ideas and trying to come up with something clever. Finally, I suggested "Miss Scarlet Rose."

That's how Rosie came to be with us. Now we had three therapy dogs.

I was supposed to start treatment in a few days, so I went with Mom to the hospital where Dad was recovering from his latest graft surgery to repair his leg—unfortunately he was in a hospital on the other side of the river from the hospital where I was being treated. Before we walked into the ICU, Mom drilled me. "OK, now don't mention anything about Rosie. We still have to figure out what to do about her before Dad comes home," she said.

"Right," I said. "Be cool. Be cool." Of course, in the end, I was the one who blew it. We were sitting with him in his aquarium room, and he was hooked up to all sorts of tubes and monitors. I imagine this is what I looked like when I had been in intensive care, which was not good. "Hey, Dad," I said, "do you know that if you hold your breath for as long as you can, the lines on your monitor go way down, and if you hold it long enough, a buzzer will go off?"

"I know." He grinned. "I can't get them low enough to set off anything, and that's probably good, but I can get them pretty low. So how's the Boo?"

"Oh, you know, I went to school, and rode Misty, and then I took Sandy and Sassy and Rosie for a walk, and—" I caught myself. Mom looked at me sharply. I stopped talking instantly, frozen. But Dad doesn't miss much.

"Rosie? Who's Rosie?"

Mom and I looked at each other. She signed and gestured for me to follow through. "Go on. Tell him." I groaned inwardly. Time to bite the bullet.

"Uh, Rosie is…" I paused, afraid. *Oh just say it, you big wiener. Say it and get it over with.* "Rosie is my puppy. My friend gave me a puppy for my birthday."

Dad didn't say anything. So I blundered on.

"She's really cute. She already weighs thirty pounds and she's only three months old!" Yeah. Wrong thing to say, Lindsey. I looked up at his monitor, where his heart rate and BP were climbing. Steadily.

Dad didn't move.

"Dad?" I asked.

"Did you know about this?" he asked Mom.

"No! They just showed up with this puppy! What was I supposed to do? Tell them to take it back?"

"Well…yeah. You could have. Two dogs aren't enough?"

"*Wes*! It was a birthday gift to *Lindsey*, not us."

"Well, we're the one's who are going to pay for it, aren't we?" Oh, great. Here we go. It looked like Rosie was going back where she came from. At least Dad realized he had no control over the situation in his current position. "We'll figure out what to do when I get home." I left that day figuring that by the time I came home from my first cycle of chemo, Rosie would be long gone.

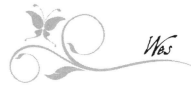

The Zofran worked so amazingly that she was able to keep food down. I thought, What a fabulous advancement this is. Everything about it is just better.

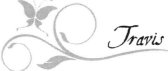

I had to bide my time. There were a lot of hours to while away. I would follow the Nintendo cart around to different rooms and make friends with whoever was playing. But the best part about being at Doernbecher was going into the playroom and making paper airplanes out of the construction paper. We were pretty high up, on the fourteenth floor, so we would open the windows and see how far the planes would fly. Then one day, they put in new childproof windows, and my paper airplane flights were over forever.

For every chemo cycle, which would last between three and five days, depending on which drug or drugs I was to receive, I would start out in the peds hem/onc clinic with Dr. Wolff. Kaylee would access my port, draw blood, and start me on fluids—you always got at least an hour of fluids before they started running the drug itself in—what is tantamount to a sophisticated cellular poison—then Dr. Wolff would come in to "take a peek," as he liked to say. We'd go through the normal physical exam routine, and when they were satisfied, they'd send me off to 14A. Mom and I would take the big faux Louis Vuitton bag and walk over the sky bridge to the South Hospital and check in with Karen. More often than not, they would put me in the same single room where I had recovered from surgery. It soon came to be known as "Lindsey's Teen Suite." We joked about how it should have a plaque on the wall bearing my name instead of a room number.

They were using different agents this time. Instead of vincristine, dactinomycin, and doxorubicin, I was getting Cytoxan (cyclophosphamide), VP-16 (etoposide), and carboplatin. The Cytoxan and the VP-16 came together, along with another drug called Mesna. The Mesna was intended to form a protective coating in the urinary tract because cyclophosphamide is known to deteriorate the tissue there and cause bleeding. Consequently, I also learned how to pee in a "hat." Every time I checked in, Karen would write my name in thick black marker on this white plastic cylinder that had flat, wing-like protrusions on either side. It was marked with units like a measuring cup. The first day, she brought it in with much fanfare and said, "Here's your hat!"

"My hat?" I looked at it. It vaguely resembled a combination of those old three-cornered hats they used to wear back during the Revolutionary War, and Abe Lincoln's hat. "What is it for?"

"You get to pee in the hat. Every time you pee, Dr. Wolff wants you peein' in here."

"What? Why?" It was funny. I smiled at her. Was this for real? I was looking for a punch line in what she said and couldn't find one. *Every* time I peed they wanted a sample? That's a lot of pee when you're hooked up to a fire hose of an IV.

"I'll be checking it periodically for blood. We dip a little strip in it, and it turns color if there's blood in there. The Cytoxan can cause you to bleed, and obviously, we don't want that."

"Oh. OK." Sure. I'll pee wherever they want me to pee.

"Or you can use the commode," she offered. "Would you rather?"

I thought about it. No way. The idea of sitting on this thing that looked like a regular metal chair with little wheels and *peeing* kinda weirded me out. I said, "Uhh…no, I don't think so." It's not like I had anything else to do. I could afford to walk between my room and the bathroom. "All right," Karen said as she walked out the room, "It'll be in the bathroom. Just find it, slide it under the seat in the bowl and pee away!"

She always cracked me up.

Awhile later, she returned and injected some clear liquid into the IV drip.

"What's that?" I asked. I always wanted to know what they were putting in there, so I could be prepared if it was going to make me sick, or make sure they weren't giving me the wrong thing.

I supposed it *was* pretty easy to get kids mixed up—we were all bald and pale, anyway.

"This is your Zofran. Wouldn't want to start chemo without it!" Ah, the Zofran. The rumored manna from heaven. I was interested to see how it worked—*if* it worked. Part of me still refused to accept the idea of chemo without nausea.

"How does it work? Like the Benadryl?" I asked.

"Nope. It won't put you to sleep. It blocks special receptors in your stomach and esophagus and basically prevents your brain from noticing the nausea." That sounded pretty cool. "It's not perfect," she continued, "it can't block them all, but you should feel pretty good." She pressed a series of buttons on the blue pump. "We'll run this over a half hour. Then we'll do another half hour of plain old fluids. Then we'll start your chemo."

"So I get Zofran an hour before chemo? Every time?" I asked.

"Yeah, it only works if the first dose is given before the chemo. Then you have it every four hours afterward." This was exactly the reason I was opting for treatment in the hospital instead of as an outpatient: to make sure I was getting my Zofran every four hours. I didn't even want to take a chance that it would run out and stop working and I'd have to go through the rest of the chemo cycle without it.

"Oh, right," she remembered as she left, "I'll get you some menus, too, for today and tomorrow." Oh, great. More hospital food. Hurrah. Maybe Dominos would deliver to 14A…turns out, they do.

I was working on what foods would be the least of all evils when Karen came back with the chemo. "This you?" she asked as she showed me the label on the bag. It said cyclophosphamide and below that a bunch of numbers, my birth date, and my name.

"Yep. That's me," I said. She pulled the tube from the bag of saline and plugged into the chemo. She beeped the buttons on the pump and was making some notes when I said, "Karen, I don't want any of this food. I mean, 'London Broil'? I mean, I don't even know for sure what that *is*."

"Just write in what you want then. There are some things they'll give you if you write it in. Especially at breakfast, you can get other cereals and stuff." Now *that* was a good idea. I'd stock up again on the little cereals so I didn't have to eat the other stuff. What I really wanted was a big croissant with deli turkey, a little mayonnaise, mustard, lettuce, Tillamook cheddar, and tomato. That was my big thing lately. I wondered if they could come through for me. In the end, I went with a hamburger and fries for dinner. How could they mess that up, right?

When I finished with my menus, I sat back in the bed and watched the chemo drip into the IV line and creep its way toward my port. As the yellow liquid inched closer and closer, I thought, *This is it. This is real. I'm doing chemo again.* And it hit me all of a sudden how surreal it all felt. This was my life? The things that I had done in the past year and a half were the types of things you only read about in magazines (and I had). Everyone was always so impressed and called me "brave," and I always thought, *But I'm not. I just do what they tell me to do. You'd do it, too, if you didn't have a choice.* There was nothing special about me; I was just following directions. You would, too, if you had to. Besides, if *I* could do it, then it must not be *that* hard.

I pressed the call button wrapped around the rail on my bed and someone crackled on the speaker. "I have my menus ready," I said loudly. I received a squelch of acknowledgement and a few minutes later Karen appeared and took them away. I passed the day by talking to Mom, watching cable, reading, drawing, and doing homework. By that evening, I felt mildly nauseous but not distractingly so, and it was definitely tolerable. My dinner showed up, but it reeked of grease so badly that I made Mom take it away. I ended up throwing up once that night, and it was the only time I vomited that whole week.

Since I was stable and used to the idea of getting chemo, it wasn't necessary for Mom or anyone to stay with me overnight. People would come up and hang out during the day: Mom, Holly, Jeanna, whomever, but at night it was just me and Denise, my favorite swing-shift nurse, and then me and whomever the grave-yard nurse was.

Once, Mom and I were sitting in the room and someone knocked on the door. We let them in, and it was pet therapy. An older lady had brought her lap-sized poodle. It was squeaky clean and let itself be handled like a curly ragdoll. She'd put it on the bed and it just lay there and let us pet it while it wagged its shaggy stump of a tail. It wore a little vest emblazoned with the name of the pet therapy organization. She put it on the floor and it did a few tricks. This experience gave Mom an idea, and the next time I was in for a cycle, she scrubbed Sandy Dunes and tied a bright yellow kerchief around her neck, put her in her crate, and carried her up to the ward.

"Of course, I didn't think about this until right now," she said as she came in the room and shut the door behind her, "but I wonder if it's OK that I have Sandy Dunes with me."

"I don't know," I said. It was later in the evening, and Denise was my nurse at the moment. We called her. When she came in, we asked about Sandy Dunes.

"Since she's not a certified pet therapy dog, she can't be around anyone else, but there's probably no reason why she can't be in here with you. We should talk to Dr. Wolff to be sure." Dr. Wolff ended up giving the green light to brief occasional visits from Sandy Dunes, but she was not allowed to come into contact with anyone else, just in case another child caused her to snap or something. And on her trips in and out of the ward, other kids would see her and say, "That's a really cool dog," or "Look at that! It's a circus dog!"

When she came, she would sit on the bed for a while with me, and if I could stand to have a tray of food in my room I'd give her bits and pieces; but most of the time, I asked Karen and Denise to not even bother with the food. They left it on the cart and it went back where it came from. When it was time for the food cart to come up to the ward, they were even considerate enough to close the door for me so the greasy smell that permeated the entire ward wouldn't enter my room.

Fairly early every morning, the group of students would tour the rooms and wake me up for a "how-are-you-sleeping" check. Dr. Wolff would show up a little later in the morning, sometimes alone, sometimes accompanied by his cohorts Norman and Stein. I finally asked him about the test he was going to give me, to which he responded, "Are you ready for it?" I was as ready as I would ever be. He left and returned later with a piece of paper on which were scribbled five questions. I set about answering them, and when he returned later he graded it. I clenched my teeth in anticipation.

"Five for five," he announced, putting it back on my bed-table. I was relieved and impressed with myself, and suddenly eager to know more. So a few weeks later I went with Holly and her mom to the famous Powell's bookstore in Portland. I eventually found the medical section and stumbled across a medical dictionary/encyclopedia. It was about as thick as the Bible we had at home, and it was fascinating. I spent the whole trip reading it, and neglected to get any of the books I'd initially set out for. When they came looking for me when it was time to leave, I checked the price of the book: forty-five dollars. Crestfallen, I replaced it on the shelf and followed Holly out of the store, still absorbed in the world of polysyllabic mystery words and insanely detailed drawings of the human body. I was in love.

The night after I came home from the first cycle of treatment, I faced my first Neupogen injection. I fetched one of the tiny one-cc bottles from the fridge and set it on the table. They had little caps that said, "Flip Off," a phrase which both Holly and I found highly amusing, and were sure to use in public at all possible opportunities. In my room I kept a stockpile of one-cc syringes, tiny 27½-gauge needles, a sharps box for the used needles and a large supply of alcohol pads. I sat down at the table, screwed the needle into the syringe, and popped the top. I swabbed the rubber with an alcohol pad, pulled the plunger all the way back on the syringe, inserted the needle, injected the air, drew one cc of the fluid out, tapped the bubbles, and carefully recapped the needle by setting it down and scooting it back into the cap. I took my trusty ice pack from the freezer and proceeded to try and numb the skin on my thigh. I never quite got the results I really wanted. Instead of dead numbness, it always felt stingingly cold. Then I'd swab the skin with an alcohol pad, uncap the needle again, and go through the mental battle with myself over injecting/not injecting. My dichotomous inner dialogue always went something like this:

OK, here we go. On three, then push it fast. One, two, thr—

No! Don't do it! What, are you crazy? Why do you want to hurt yourself?

Oh, for God's sake, just do it, Loser. You know you have to. You can put up with the sting, you big pansy.

Oh, please, it's about so much more than the sting.

OK, seriously now. I don't want to sit here forever agonizing over one measly milliliter. It's literally a drop in the bucket! Just do it!

Round and round with myself I would go. Do it. Don't do it. Do it. Don't do it. Finally, I'd have myself so psyched out that I wouldn't do anything and I'd end up sitting there forever. In the end, it always went in, and I always hated doing it. Sometimes the it took so long to actually do the injection that the medicine had warmed up, and I found out the hard way that it doesn't work anymore when it's at room temperature. As I cleaned up all my paraphernalia, and dumped the needles in a sharps box, I thanked God I wasn't a diabetic, and I knew that I would *never* get into drugs.

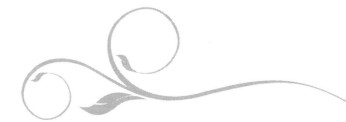

In late October, the parent's board at my school met to discuss the logistics of sending all the eighth graders to Washington, DC. Which tour company to use, where to stay, how much it would cost, how the students would raise the money, and how the money would be distributed. They also voted that it was unrealistic to think I'd be able to go out fundraising and decided to split the pot evenly amongst all the students, including me. Looks like I *was* going to get to go to DC after all.

About a week after my first cycle of cyclophosphamide and etoposide, I awoke in the middle of the night absolutely freezing. I shivered so uncontrollably I felt like I was seizing. My room was on the northeast corner of the house and had always been colder than all the other rooms, but this was ridiculous. I curled myself up in a ball as tight as I could, and still warmth eluded me. I didn't want to get up and take a shower, considering that it was the wee hours of the morning. I got up quickly, dug out several blankets from the hall closet, and piled them on my bed. I also plugged in the electric blanket that normally was on my bed and switched it on. Within an hour I felt a little warmer and went back to sleep, huddled in a tight ball.

The next morning I awoke and dopily got out of bed. As soon as I stood up, my head felt strange and achy. I was still freezing, and all I wanted to do was go back to sleep. It felt like someone was rubbing over my whole body with Velcro. Everything was prickly. I felt like I was getting the flu.

I went to find Mom, who was cleaning. She felt my head and said, "Good God, Lindsey, you're on fire. I'm getting the thermometer." My temperature ended up being well over 101. Mom called Dr. Wolff, who ordered me to 14A within the hour. I showed up at the nurse's station feeling worse than ever, clothed in several layers, and still shaking with cold. They put me in an isolation room right near the station. It was like a normal private room, except outside there was a special washing/gowning area that had doors like the aquarium rooms in the ICU. They taped a yellow sign to my door that said:

```
DANGER
ALL PERSONNEL MUST WEAR:
    GOWN   GLOVES
    MASK   EYEWEAR
```

Except someone had crossed out "eyewear," "gloves," and "gown." I couldn't stop shivering. Someone rolled in the scale, blood pressure machine, and those disposable Tempa-Dot thermometers. She weighed me, took my BP and temperature, and left, saying that IV therapy would be up as soon as possible to access my port. They brought in a commode and said I shouldn't go out to the bathroom but that I had to stay in here. Someone came in and draped a bright yellow disposable stethoscope on my IV pole. Eventually, Dr. Wolff showed up to "take a peek."

"Been a little cold, lately?" he asked while he looked over my chart. I shivered in response. He listened to me breathe and said, "All right, sounds like there's quite a bit of crackling in there. Let's get some blood cultures. Are you accessed yet?"

"No," I responded. "They said someone was coming soon. What does crackling mean?"

"It usually means a little pneumonia, but we need to do cultures to be sure. Oh, here they are. I'll be back."

IV therapy came in and prepped me for access. When they were finished, a nurse came in and drew for my cultures. She screwed one of the most enormous syringes I'd ever seen to the little hose coming out of my port and pulled back on the plunger. Blood came gushing out, filling the syringe. I watched it in awe, thinking, *Jeez, leave some for me.* She took several of those syringes and left me with a little cup full of liquid Tylenol.

"It works faster than the pills," she said as she left. I drank it and buried myself under as many blankets as they would give me. Within the hour, I started feeling warm, and I began peeling the blankets off, one by one, until I felt normal again. When my bag of water was empty, the pump started its obnoxious beep, so I pressed the button. Karen's voice crackled out.

"What you doin' here, girl?"

"Kar-en!" I shouted, singsong. "I'm beeping!"

"OK, I'll be in. Just a sec." She showed up a few minutes later, masked, with a fresh bag of saline and a big syringe of yellow stuff. "It's been crazy today," she said, "I haven't been able to get to you yet; we had to have one of the night nurses stay to help out for a while." She changed out the bag.

"What's that?" I asked, pointing to the syringe.

"That," she said, sitting down, "is vancomycin. Antibiotic. We're gonna load you up and get rid of this infection. It'll be a nice excuse for me to sit down for a second. It has to be pushed nice and slow."

"Why so slow?" I asked.

"Because sometimes people can react to it. It makes you hot and you turn red. We call it 'redneck syndrome.'"

Ha, redneck syndrome. That's rich, I thought. It's funny 'cause I live on a farm.

"But don't worry," she said, "I haven't had that happen yet." She screwed the syringe into the little tube and pushed the plunger a little. We waited a few minutes, while Karen and Mom had a conversation. She pushed again. We waited. Pushed again. Waited. She pushed the fourth time— by this time we were less than a third of the way through the total volume in the syringe—and at first it was fine; then I could feel the warmth in my body spreading. I don't know if she slipped and pushed too much or if we didn't wait long enough between pushes, but within seconds I felt as though someone had drenched me in gasoline from the chest up and set a match to me. I was on fire, and it was excruciating. Mom ran to the sink and soaked a cloth in cold water, and pressed it against my head while Karen dropped the syringe on the bed and ran. She dashed back in about thirty seconds later, a small syringe of clear liquid in her hand. "Benadryl," she said flatly as she tore off the cap and jammed the needle into the Y-junction on my line almost right up against my port and pushed the entire contents of the syringe in a flash. I had enough time to watch it go in and look up at her before I felt my whole body give an intense shudder; then I fell back, dead asleep.

Several hours later I woke up. Mom was still there. I still had the cool cloth on my forehead. "Took a little nappie, there, didn't ya, Booie?" she asked. I was groggy and slow. "You remember you reacted to the antibiotic? You got redneck syndrome. It was pretty amazing. You turned lobster red right before our eyes. Karen decided we won't push the meds anymore. She made sure everyone knows you get your vanco in the drip."

I had redneck syndrome. Now that the pain was gone, it was hilarious.

After four days of combined antibiotics vancomycin and ceftazidime, I was off the Tylenol and had no crackling in my lungs. They let me go home. I had to see Dr. Wolff a couple times every week but otherwise was looking at having two weeks off before the next cycle. I went to school, took care of my horse, gave myself shots of G-CSF—I used an ice pack to numb my leg every time, and I was such a chicken it would take me a half hour or more to do it every night—and took my Septra twice a day, three days out of the seven. After much scheming and nagging, I was finally able to convince Dr. Wolff that I shouldn't have to take the Septra while I was in for a cycle of chemo, not an easy task, and that the last thing they did before they de-accessed my port was to run the G-CSF through the line, so I didn't have to take a shot that day. I couldn't believe my luck that they were letting me get away with this stuff.

I was on day seventeen when Halloween rolled around. I was praying that my hair wouldn't start to go until afterward because I was supposed to go to a party at a friend's house. I wanted to be a hippie, and *everyone* knows hippies have long hair. I got away with all that, too, and enjoyed a night of friends and junk food. It was more fun than humans should have.

The next morning, the first clumps of hair fell out.

Mom decided that I should have a wig for certain occasions where I might be likely to freak people out if I showed up hairless, or for occasions that demanded some sort of semiformal dress. This time, we opted for a synthetic wig and went to a store in SE Portland near the Hawthorne district. We went as soon as my hair started to go so that I could get used to the wig before everything was gone. They told us that synthetic hair lasts about three months before it starts to break down a little and look fake, and that we could wash it and comb it just like normal hair. It would be light-weight enough that it wouldn't have to be pinned into place, and the cap was elastic, thus eliminating the need for tape. After we selected the wig and paid for it (significantly less than the human hair wig—under one hundred dollars), I opted for them to shave my head.

"Just get it over with and then I won't have to watch it fall out," I demanded. The lady nodded and grabbed the hair clippers. She clicked it on, and I felt the vibrations on my scalp as it buzzed away my shoulder-length locks, one strip at a time. It was extremely unsettling to watch my hair being stripped from my head, falling from my shoulders into a big pile on the floor. I could feel the tears welling up in my eyes but forced them back, biting my tongue and commanding myself not to cry. It would have been easy to start shrieking, knowing that watching my hair fall was the final estab-lishment that this was real, that there would be no waking up from this. The next morning as I stood in the shower feeling the odd sensation of water bouncing off my scalp, I felt that losing it all in one fell swoop might have been less trouble, but it was certainly no less troubling.

I opted to wear the wig home, since I hadn't thought of bring-ing a hat to keep me warm. As I looked at myself in the mirror, straightening my "hair" on my head, I thought it looked phony. To me, it didn't matter how expensive or inexpensive the wig was; it was going to be fake. I all of a sudden had bangs—which I hadn't had since fourth grade—and soon, I wouldn't have brows or lashes to reinforce the illusion. The general public is easy to fool, though.

The beginning of the second cycle was due to begin on a Friday afternoon. As Mom and I were en route to the hospital, Sharon called the car phone to invite me over because her niece and nephew–my friends–were staying the night with her. Mom handed the phone to me. "Sorry, Sharon, I'm going in for chemo right now." I was hugely disappointed, missing a sleepover for stupid chemo!

"Oh, punkin, that's too bad. Is it just for one day? Maybe you could come tomorrow."

"No, I'll be in for the next five days."

"OK, just a minute." I could hear her cover the phone with her hand and say something to someone behind her. Then everyone was on the phone at once trying to convince me to come over. It made me angry that any normal kid only had one barrier to overcome concerning sleepovers: parental approval. I had the additional barrier of treatment schedules. Funny thing was, the parental approval part was rarely a problem. I was able to get them off the phone with a "maybe next time" and I hung up feeling very cheated.

When we got to the clinic, Dr. Wolff saw us right away. Since I was the last patient on the schedule that day, he sat down and chatted for a while. Sometimes, we caught him on a chatty day and he'd sit and tell story after story. Especially track and field stories. He told us about the time he answered an ad for a guy who was custom making track shoes, and he showed up at this house to buy the shoes. Turns out, it was Bill Bowerman making those shoes in his garage, before the days of Nike. Those storytelling days are good days, because Wolff is given to loud laughter. It's good to see that in a guy who has a very serious job. Finally, he stood up and asked if I was ready for Kaylee to access my port.

"I guess," I said sulkily.

"What's with that?" he asked, hands in his pockets.

"Nothing," I said. I looked at Mom. She shrugged at me. "Go ahead. Tell him." I looked back at the Wolff-man. Oh, what the hell. "Can we do treatment Monday through Friday?" I asked hopefully. "Then I maybe can have weekends with my friends?" I added. I clenched my teeth. There was *no way* he would go for this. I'd already talked him into inpatient treatments, G-CSF in the port, *and* I was getting away with *not* taking Septra during my inpatient stays. I squinted, waiting for the big veto, but he surprised me, as he sometimes does.

He shrugged with his hands in his short lab coat. "Sure. Why not?"

I was shocked. "Really?" OK seriously, was I going to get away with *all* of my demands? He looked at his watch. "In fact, why don't you go right now, and we'll see you Monday." I looked at him, mouth open. I looked at Mom, mouth open. I couldn't believe I'd almost gotten away with this. Was I...*in charge?*

"OK, Lindsey, let's go. I gotta get you out to Sharon's now." And now Mom was willing to drive all the way back out there. I cheered inwardly and would've given Dr. Wolff a big hug, but I didn't know if that was appropriate. Are patients supposed to hug their doctors? Wolff didn't seem like the hugsy type.

In the car, I wondered aloud why Dr. Wolff was being so flexible with my treatment schedule. "I thought all this stuff was all figured out beforehand by the study. I thought we had to stick to a specific schedule in order for it to work."

"Oh, I think he's probably giving you an exception since he believes we're just doing this for backup anyway," Mom posited. I had a fantastic weekend with my friends and was completely happy to go "pay my dues" for the following week.

During the next cycle, when I saw Dr. Wolff on one of his morning visits, I asked him if I could see his medical dictionary. He smiled his patient, passive smile and agreed to bring it that evening when he returned for rounds. When he did, it looked like a very old and battered copy, and was significantly less reader-friendly than the one I'd found at Powell's. But I leafed through it to pass the time. I was in a double room, so I had to share the TV, and I needed something to do.

When he came back the next morning, I asked if I could read my charts. He paused for a while, looking at the floor and finally shrugged, saying, "I don't see why not. They technically *are* yours." Hurrah! Then he added, wagging a finger at me, "But I don't want you reading it by yourself because you won't understand a lot of it. I'll send someone in with it later today, and he or she will sit with you and go through it." Later that day, a slightly disgruntled looking young man in a mid-length lab coat came in with my file that was easily as thick as the dictionary I'd been reading. It was so huge, I couldn't get far at all, but we did go through both of my surgical reports and a few daily notes—which were written in almost completely indecipherable chicken scratch. I learned about the inferior vena cava–the major vein that returns blood from the body to the heart–different types of surgical silk used for stitches, electrocautery, and the different positions they put people in for surgeries. For my first one, I was in the "supine" position—flat on my back—but for my second, they put me on my left side, with my right arm over my head. I learned that my first operation was called a radical left nephrectomy. I guessed that "radical" in this case meant "whole" or "complete," instead of "awesome." It was very interesting, but before long I was tired and he had to go on rounds again, so show-and-tell with the chart was over for the day.

I lay there, drifting off, thinking about the information I'd just read and how intriguing it was. Most of my life I had wanted to study veterinary medicine, specifically large animals, but my interest had been piqued with this information about my disease. I was fascinating! Perhaps I would go into human medicine. After all, humans are big animals, too. At the end of the year my school had a science fair. Everyone had to do a project, so I decided I would do mine on me. Feeling very satisfied with myself, I went to sleep.

The Zofran seemed to be working. I would feel slightly off the first night, but the rest of the week I would be fine. It didn't do anything for the food aversions, however. I knew exactly which hours of the day the door needed to be closed so that I might spare myself the wafting stink of food and grease. The very idea of my once favorite turkey croissant was enough to make me green. Mostly, I lived off of small boxes of cereal that I would hoard from my breakfast trays, sending all the others back to the kitchen. The only thing I ever wanted was Taco Bell nachos, which Mom would take me to get right after leaving the hospital each time. Of course, I found out later that there was someone keeping tabs on how many trays come back to the hospital kitchens full of food, and which patients they were supposed to go to. So periodically I would get a visit from some dietician trying to find out why I wasn't eating. I would look at her and marvel at her stupidity, trying to refrain myself from shouting, "Hello! I'm on chemo! It's called *anorexia*, and it's a side effect. I don't want your crap food because it smells bad. Now leave me alone with my cereal boxes and go bug the real anorexics. They're the ones you should be worrying about!"

Instead, I would tell her that the food smelled bad and asked them to not even bring it in. "You know you can write in pretty much anything you want, right?" she asked. *Yes, I know that, thank you.* I was a pro at this. I knew how things worked. I wanted to put my arm around her shoulders, walk her out of the room, and say, "Pumpkin. Sweetheart. I am the least of your problems. You might want to start with firing your chef and finding another company that has more experience in preparing food for the masses. Perhaps a cruise line will suit your needs." Instead I sat there and let her patronize me about how important it was to eat, needing to keep my strength up, food helping to heal me, blah, blah, blah-dee blah. I'd usually just tune her out until she asked another question.

"If you could have anything you wanted to eat right now, what would it be?" she asked, clipboard at the ready.

"Nothing," I said.

"Come on, really. Anything in the world."

I stared at her. Seriously, what did I have to do to get this chick to leave me alone? Just name a food. Tell her anything so she'll leave, and then whatever it is she sends to you, you can send back to her.

"Fine. Fruit salad."

"OK, good. Good. Fruit salad. That's easy. We'll send one right up." And she left. Later that day, a fruit salad did show up, and since it didn't smell, I actually ate it.

Kaylee

Kids get cancer, and somebody has to take care of them. When I first got the job, I thought, This has to be the worst job in the world, but I took it because I needed a job. Little did I know I would absolutely love it. I think that it's a privilege and that you become a part of someone's family in a time of complete and utter horror and trauma. To watch your child be put through all kinds of horrible medications and pokes and nausea and the whole thing, has got to be the worst experience of a parent's life. Especially if it happens again a second time. The nurse becomes a very trusted person, a source of comfort. It's a privilege to take care of these families. That's what carried me through. My skills are able to help a child have a better day. That's how I was able to go to work and do my job every day.

A few days after the second cycle of chemo, I saw Dr. Wolff once; and a couple days after that, I found myself back in my suite, again in isolation. I woke up one morning shivering with a major fever, and sure enough my lungs were crackling away. They took another gallon of blood for cultures, gave me Tylenol, and sent the antibiotics perking through my veins. I figured this would become routine: in for a week, out for a week, in for a week, out for two or three weeks, in for a week, etc. It would be like this until May, and here we were, only in November.

I was sitting around on my bed one day, watching the construction outside, when Holly came in to visit. We talked for a while, and then she went over to the window and opened it, saying, "I bet we could spit on someone from way up here!"

As soon as I saw the window open, I wondered if that was a good idea, but I still laughed at her idea of trying to spit on someone from fourteen stories up. We heard the door open and both looked at Dr. Wolff standing in the doorway.

"Shut that window, *now!*" he commanded. Holly slammed it shut. I shrank back in disbelief. I'd never heard Dr. Wolff raise his voice like that. He glared at both of us.

"Did you know that this room has a special ventilation system to keep it clean? And now you've contaminated it?"

We both looked at him. "No," I said. "Really? It does?"

"It *did*. Now you have contaminants from that construction site out there blowing around in here."

I was suddenly scared. Was my infection going to get worse now? Just because we'd opened a lousy *window*? I didn't really know we were doing anything wrong; otherwise I would have stopped Holly. Why was the window even open-able in the first place?

"Sorry, Wolffy," Holly said quietly, sheepishly.

"It's OK for now. Just don't ever do it again. When in doubt, do *not* open the windows." He turned his attention to me. "Have you left this room yet?"

"No," I said, confused as to why he'd ask when the sign on the door said, "Patient is to remain in isolation."

"I want you to go out of the room, OK? Don't worry. Wear a mask and wash your hands frequently, and you'll be fine. I'd rather you go down to the school session or something than stay in here all the time."

I was suddenly confused. We'd just gotten in trouble for contaminating the special ventilation system, and now he *wanted* me to leave the room and go hang around the other sick people? Crazy.

After he left, Holly said, "Oh, check this out!" and she gave me a thin strip of…something. Was it plastic? Was it metal? I thought it was metal but wasn't sure. It was a silvery iridescent color. She showed me how it worked. "You put it down on your wrist, flat side against your skin, and then tap your wrist with it." I did what she said. With a sharp *slap!* the thin metal strip wrapped itself around my wrist.

"It's a slap-bracelet!" she announced gleefully. I pulled it off, straightened it out, and did it again. It slapped around my wrist. There was something oddly satisfying about hearing that painless yet distinctly loud slap. The slap-bracelet passed many hours. It always curled perfectly around and always straightened perfectly out again. I haven't seen them anywhere since.

Being in the hospital so much caused me to miss 122½ days of school that year. It was cramping my style because I had managed to get into the advanced English class and Algebra I. I didn't want to lose that English class because the few of us were permitted to study independently in the hall, which of course meant an hour of unsupervised yakking. But continued allowance into the advanced English group was contingent on my performance on the teacher's dreaded proficiency tests, and it was getting harder and harder to keep up. As for algebra, my workload had been lessened considerably. I only had to do every fifth problem, but missing out on the lecture portion of class was killing me. Luckily, there were a few teachers on the ward, and every day from nine a.m. to twelve p.m. school was in session in the playroom. I would go down there to get help on my algebra and work on my other homework. I would also pass the time on the ward with one of the two computers, playing the Oregon Trail game, doing crosswords, and working on math. Conversely, at home, my parents were unable to help me effectively with homework, so Dad called one of his brothers who had gone to college and earned a degree in biology to help me out with math. I worked hard enough to squeak by, but missing so much school was adding up.

After my third round of chemo and pneumonia, I was ordered to get my first transfusion. I didn't want a transfusion. I felt somehow weaker or more defeated that I had to get someone else's blood to get through this. We were in the clinic, and Dr. Wolff came in saying my counts were so low he didn't want to send me home without blood. He had some paperwork for us to read so we could understand how the transfusions worked and the risks. I knew about HIV and AIDS, and I wanted to know how easily I could get it.

"Everyone wants to know about HIV risk, but it really isn't that big at all. You have a much higher risk of getting Hepatitis-C from it," Dr. Wolff said. *Oh, yeah, thanks Wolffy, that makes me feel better.* I looked at Mom, who was concerned since a good friend of hers—a health inspector—had died from Hepatitis-A several years before. Dr. Wolff went through all the paperwork with us, and we all signed, Mom, Dad, and me. Soon, a little bag of blood showed up and they plugged me in. There were different types of blood I could get: red cells, platelets, whole blood, but never white cells. Today was a red cell day, and after the transfusion was over, I felt pretty good. Gotta love that oxygen flowin' through your veins.

Periodically, through the rest of my treatment protocol, I'd receive various blood products. One day in particular, my labs came back indicating that my platelets had dropped to a measly 14,000 (in a normal person they should be 130,000 and up) and Wolff looked at me wryly, handed the printout over and said, "Oh, how 'bout some platelets today?"

Linda

They had to use different chemo agents this time, to make it stronger. We knew going into it that the side effects were going to be more brutal. By this time, I knew what to look for, so I could identify problems immediately and get her to Dr. Wolff. And there was a sense of relief when I did get her there because I knew she was in the best of hands.

We were also given an option to harvest her bone marrow so if she should relapse again, we could go straight into a bone marrow transplant. It was like, "Yeah. There is no doubt. We're doing that."

By the New Year, I'd had several rounds of chemo in the hospital, and each one was followed by a bout with pneumonia and still more time in the hospital. It was starting to make me a little stir-crazy, so when Dr. Wolff proposed that I go off treatment for the entire month of February, I was fine with that.

"We want to have some insurance so that if you should ever relapse with Wilms we're ready for it. So, I'm going to take you off treatment and let your counts recover for a month. Then, at the end of the month we want to harvest your marrow. We'll put it in a freezer and it will be available for the next ten years, just in case." He looked at me expectantly as if I was going to challenge his expertise.

"Sounds good." I shrugged.

"I will be handing you over to Dr. Stein's care for February to monitor you and decide when we'll do the harvest," he said. Now *that* I felt like challenging. I didn't like her. She didn't exactly have the greatest bedside manner, and I didn't care how smart she was, I didn't like her. I didn't say as much to Dr. Wolff, because I knew he would never make a bad decision about me, but I suddenly wanted to be back *on* treatment as quickly as possible, since that meant I could have my Wolff back.

"Is a bone marrow transplant the same as an organ transplant as far as rejection goes?" Dad asked. He still had his giant cast and had to wear shorts all the time. Before he answered, Dr. Wolff sat down in the only available chair in the room—a toddler sized wooden chair, that he often remarked was his favorite chair in the whole clinic.

"It is preferable to use the patient's own bone marrow because the risk of rejection is less, yes," Dr. Wolff responded. I watched him. It was comical to listen to him talk about such important issues when he was sitting in a child-sized chair.

In the meantime, before chemo-vacation, I had another cycle to get through. I went to the clinic, as usual. Saw Dr. Wolff, as usual, and Kaylee accessed me, as usual. As she was prepping the port site, cleaning it with Betadine, she said, "Oh, no, you have such a pretty bra…I'd hate to get Betadine all over it. Even though it'll probably wash out…still…" I looked down at my bra. I hadn't thought it was particularly beautiful, but maybe it was compared to the other thirteen-year-olds in the clinic. It was a plain flesh color and had some lace on the top of the cup.

"I don't care if you get Betadine on it." She rolled the cup down as far as she could and proceeded to finish prepping the site. After the needle was in, she tried to flush the line with saline, but it wouldn't move.

"It's not…flushing," she said, frowning. She pulled the needle and replaced it, pressing harder. Still, the line wouldn't flush. "Oh, I hope your port hasn't moved," she thought aloud.

"They can move?" I exclaimed, slightly panicked, "Moved where? What do you mean?"

"Sometimes they can move out of their vessel and then they won't work anymore." Oh, God, what if it'd moved? We'd be back to the butterflies and that would suck. She quit trying to flush the line and thought for a second. "Hang on," she said as she left the room. She came back with a new tray and started completely over. As she was swabbing the Betadine, she said, "Let's try a longer needle. That one was a half-incher. Let's try a three-fourths." Yes, let's. Lo and behold, it worked. I heaved a sigh of relief. That port was the best thing about this whole process–I didn't want to lose it. "Good," she said. "I'll put a note in your chart that you always have to have at least the three-fourths needle. You just have a good, deep port."

She hitched me up to a drip, and we waited for Dr. Wolff. He came in and gave me the once-over. Afterward, he said, "It's really busy on the ward right now. Last I heard, there were no open beds. Let's keep you in the clinic for a while, and we'll start your chemo. When a bed opens up, we can send you over, or we may have to send you over to eight instead."

"What's on eight?" I asked.

"That's where the adults are."

I wouldn't mind. I figured it was all the same. A room was a room; a nurse was a nurse…except that I wanted *my* nurses.

We sat in the day room for several hours, and it made me think of last time when I received all my treatments in there. There were two beds, a TV/VCR, and a portable Super Nintendo. Mom had some Chicken in a Biskit crackers in the faux Louis Vuitton bag, and they were surprisingly palatable. In the end, a bed opened up on 14A. It was a double room, and I would be next to a three-year-old who had just had brain surgery. She made the stay pretty obnoxious, but it wasn't her fault. She was on those narcotics, and I knew very well how restless and weepy you could get on those things. By the third night, I'd barely slept at all when Denise came in to change out IV bags. The little girl was sobbing and had been doing so for a couple hours, calling periodically for her mommy, who wasn't there. She was totally alone.

"You know," Denise said as she worked, "maybe you should go down to the rec room and watch some TV. If you fall asleep in there I won't wake you, but you're not supposed to fall asleep in there…" She winked at me. I took the hint and rolled Stand-ley down the hall to the rec room that was adjacent to the playroom. In it were several couches, a TV, a mini pool table, and the door to the teachers' offices. I found the remote, clicked on the TV, and lay down on the couch. Denise came in after a while with a pillow and some clean blankets.

"Why don't we lay these down on the couch so you can be on a clean blanket, OK? Here's your pillow." I took the pillow from her and stood up while she made my "bed." She reset my IV pump flow and left. I watched late night TBS Superstation, the lineup that I was already quite familiar with thanks to long nights with high fevers: *Brady Bunch, Partridge Family, Gilligan's Island, Love Boat, The Golden Girls*. But not long after I was into the *Brady Bunch*, I was out.

I awoke the next morning, wondering how long I'd stayed in there. Had I missed morning rounds? Had Dr. Wolff been to my room and I was gone? I wondered if he'd be mad that I slept in the rec room. Part of me didn't care, because I'd probably have to do it again tonight. I went back to my room, where my neighbor was finally asleep, and noticed my breakfast tray with its stock of cereals had not arrived. So it must not have been that late.

I survived a whole week living with a toddler on narcotics, and lucky for both of us, she started doing much better near the end of the week. Finally, it was almost time to go home. I thought about the idea of being back in the hospital next week with more pneumonia. It was an unpleasant thought, to say the least.

Not long after I'd begun treatment, my periods had disappeared entirely. I didn't mind it, naturally. I also didn't have to worry about shaving my legs or anything. I finally mentioned to Mom that I hadn't had a period in a couple months. She said, "I'll talk to Dr. Wolff about it when we go up tomorrow." But we didn't see Dr. Wolff the next day. For whatever reason, he wasn't in the clinic. We got Dr. Stein instead. I sat on the table while Mom told her all about what I'd said, and asked if they would ever come back. Dr. Stein responded, "It's hard to say for sure what will happen. The body will shut off nonessential processes like that when it's under duress and starving for blood. But…there is a possibility that she will always have problems with her periods. She may be infertile…so they can correct the problem with oral contraceptives." Contraceptives? They would put me on The Pill? I didn't want that. Only slutty girls took The Pill, and I didn't want my parents to think I was promiscuous.

"…Juggle the pill so you do get your periods, or juggle the pill so you don't get your periods, it would be up to you. But seeing as how she's been irradiated to the lower abdomen, and cyclophosphamide and doxorubicin have been known to cause infertility, it's just a toss up. Some people go on to have children, some people don't, but you don't really know until you try it."

So I might not have kids, huh? That didn't really bother me. I didn't even *like* kids. I thought babies were loud and annoying. I'd never received reinforcement in my life that merely staying home with the kids and being a housewife was an honorable or desirable thing to do, even though Mom had done it most of our lives. I had been groomed to get out there and live life, be a professional, do whatever I wanted, not stay home with the brood. In short, I was fine with the idea of never having kids.

Dr. Stein's words had brought up an interesting paradox, however. I felt like it was fine for me to decide that I didn't want kids and never intended to have them, but it was quite another when an outside force seemed to decide that for me. Suddenly, the choice didn't appear to be precisely mine anymore, and I wasn't sure I was secure with that—even though I'd likely choose to not reproduce.

In the meantime, I was just happy I didn't have to deal with any of it, so I pushed it all to the back of my mind and didn't revisit it for several years.

Sure enough, I came down with another fever a few days after my latest chemo dose. *This Neupogen is crap*, I thought. *It's obviously not keeping me out of the hospital, and it sucks taking it every night. What's the point?* I happened to be home alone for most of the day, so I didn't bother calling Mom at work to tell her I felt so bad. I curled in bed with a hundred blankets on me and moaned my way through headaches and a general flu-like malaise. I kept telling myself, *It'll pass. It'll pass. You don't need to go back. It'll pass.* About four o'clock that afternoon, the phone rang. I felt worse than ever, and I reached for the phone, hoping it was Mom who would come home and make me feel better. I whined a greeting into the receiver.

"Lindsey, is that you?"

I snapped fully awake. That wasn't Mom, it was Dr. Wolff. I'd have to play my cards just right to avoid isolation.

"Hi, Dr. Wolff. I feel great." I tried my best to sound normal. I thought I was pulling it off.

"Yeah, right. I highly doubt that. You have a fever?"

"I don't know." I didn't, really. I was clawing for any legitimate excuse. "I'm just really tired."

"How's your mucous?" he asked.

"My mucous?" I was puzzled.

"Yeah. You been blowing your nose? What color is your mucous?"

I *had* been blowing my nose, and it was a delightful greenish brown color. I told him.

"You should come up here, right now." It wasn't a suggestion.

"OK, but my mom isn't here. She's at work."

"Then call her. I want to see you by five thirty on Fourteen A. All right?"

"OK..." God, I did *not* want to be in isolation *again*. I did as I was told and called Mom, who raced home, picked me up, and brought me to the hospital. When I got there, Denise said, "Oh, Lindsey, you look horrible. Your suite is ready for you, though. I'll see you in there to get your vitals." I went down to my room and shook under the blanket until Denise showed up. She stuck the Tempa-Dot under my tongue, took my BP, and laid some extra blankets on the bed. "IV therapy is coming right up to access you," she said as she taped the yellow isolation sign to my door. After I was accessed, Denise came back and took the usual amounts of blood for cultures and hooked me up. Dr. Wolff showed up later and did a once over before ordering the vanco and ceftazidime and Tylenol.

"I'll be back first thing tomorrow," he said as he left. Denise came back with Tylenol and I drank it. It didn't work right away. In fact, I didn't sleep at all that night but tuned in to good ol' TBS for some classic TV entertainment. I finally started to feel comfortable again around three or four a.m., but I wasn't tired until after I saw Dr. Wolff again, looking spry in his red bow tie, early the next morning.

A large part of me loathed spending so much time alone. Physically, I had to be alone a fair amount of the time for one reason or another—I was sick, I had pneumonia, I was too tired, or there was chicken pox lurking about—but socially, I felt entirely isolated most of the time. There were few people in my age bracket who grasped what my life was really like. I certainly learned who my real friends were, and Holly was it. She was never afraid of anything, she never treated me differently, and she never distanced herself. The most beautiful part of it all was that she was a part of my life through so much of the day-to-day stuff that I felt she genuinely knew what I was going through. I found solace in her that I couldn't find elsewhere. I often wondered if the purpose of this disease was to forge and cement a friendship with her that might transcend all time and distance. But regardless of how much time we spent together, or how often she stuck up for me when people made snide comments, jokes, or just plain stared, I realized I was missing a valuable part of teen socialization.

On the other hand, I would sometimes equally loathe being around my peers. They would yammer on about their problems—bad hair days, ugly clothes, that boy doesn't like me, who asked you to the dance, etc., etc.—and I just was unable to view them as genuine problems. Hello, people! Tryin' to stay alive here, and you're worried about your *hair* frizzing? Here's the perfect solution to frizzy hair: shave it off! I'd have to hear about how my friends' parents embarrassed them all the time, and I simply could not relate. I was closer to my parents than I'd ever been, and life wouldn't be possible without their support. They never embarrassed me.

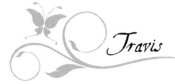

Someone in my class got chicken pox, so they were afraid that I would get it and give it to Lindsey. That would be bad. So Mom and Lindsey moved out. And it was just Dad and me at the house. We ate a lot of hot dogs.

We thought Travis had been exposed to chicken pox. We packed up and moved out of the house for the incubation period. It had to have had an effect on Travis. I wasn't there to tuck him in at night. I wasn't there during the day. I wasn't there for him. Travis didn't get the attention that Lindsey got. He became malicious in his attempts to get attention. And, being a boy, he was already a rough'n'tumble personality. I think people made an assumption that he could cope with all of this more easily because he's a boy.

Just because Mom and Dad got along with me didn't mean my brother did. He was still annoying as ever. One night, we got a call from the school saying that one of the parents reported her child, who shared a classroom with Travis, had come down with chicken pox. So Travis had been exposed. We now had a fourteen-day wait before we'd know if he was incubating the virus or if he was in the clear. That meant I had to move out. But we didn't know where I could go that I wouldn't still risk exposure to someone from the school. In the end, Sharon offered Mom and me one of the spare bedrooms in their house. They were going on vacation for a couple weeks, so we could stay there with no problem. We moved in for almost a month, and it was nice, but it's always interesting trying to get used to someone else's home. For instance, they had two Australian Shepherds who would jump into the car when we unloaded groceries, and we couldn't drag them out until we took them for a drive. So, we'd get in the car, drive to the end of the driveway, turn around, and come back. They'd happily bound from the car to the house. Another instance involved some seismic activity. Mom and I were sleeping in the guest room, and above our heads was an enormous framed child's painting of a cat. At some point in the night I woke up to something rattling around, and then *wham!* We were knocked on our heads by the painting falling on us, glass breaking everywhere.

At the end of our monthlong stay at Hotel Sharon, we were all disappointed that Travis didn't even get the virus. Essentially, we went through all that for nothing.

"All right! That's it. Next time some kid comes down with chicken pox you're going to go over and, like, *share a cup* with him," Mom told Travis.

One day while in for a routine chemo cycle, I found myself excruciatingly bored. This is unusual for me, since I'd mastered the art of blowing hours upon hours in a hospital bed. I buzzed the nurse's desk. I heard Karen's cheerful voice on the other end. "What's up, girl?"

"Karen! I...am...so...bored!"

"You know I can't medicate for *that*. I'll be in in a sec." Awhile later she came in. "Now, what are we to do with you? You want me to send in Child Life? Maybe a volunteer could come and play."

"No, I don't want to play with a stranger. How 'bout you play? You're the most fun."

"Yeah, right," she said, "You know I can't play with you. I have to work! Need the big bucks. Have you done your homework?"

"Yeah," I said dully.

"How about the computer? I could get that for you..."

No way. I was burnt out on drawing, computers, crosswords, etc. Even the slap bracelet couldn't save me now. Suddenly Karen lit up.

"Hey, get your pole, girl. Come with me."

I jumped out of bed and unplugged Stand-ley, wrapped the cord up, and followed her out the door. She walked me down the hall to the isolation rooms, knocked on the door, and motioned for me to come in with her. On the bed was a boy about my age or slightly older. He had blue eyes and was just as white and hairless as I was. I dare say he was prettier than I—he didn't appear to be retaining water like I was. Karen introduced us.

"Hey, Chris, this is Lindsey. Lindsey, this is Chris. He's about the only one on the floor in your age bracket. Maybe you two can hang out and cure each other's boredom." From outside the room, someone called for Karen to go down to room 23. "Gotta go, guys." She left. I stood there, stupidly, in the doorway, looking at him. He looked back at me. I looked at the floor.

"So...you're Chris?" I asked lamely.

"Yeah," he said quietly. I had no idea what to say. Was I supposed to *hang out* in here, or what? Just plop down on his bed and play checkers or something? This guy was a stranger. Well, we did have *one* thing in common.

"What do you have?" I asked him.

"AML," he replied.

"I have Wilms Tumor. It's kidney cancer. What's AML?" I'd never taken the time to think about other diseases besides mine. I'd always assumed that each one was similar in severity, treatment, and success rates.

"It's leukemia. They call it acute myelogenous leukemia."

"Oh," I said. Leukemia just *sounded* so much worse than cancer, having four syllables rather than two. My mind raced, trying vainly to find something else to ask him. Ideally something that would make me sound cool. Finally, I had something.

"Who's your doctor?" I was hoping he'd say Dr. Wolff, so we could swap stories.

"Dr. Stein."

"Oh," I thought, Great. Dr. Stein. How am I supposed to connect with him on that one? He probably loves her as his doctor. "I have Dr. Wolff. He's totally cool," I finished.

"Yeah, I really like Dr. Stein," he said.

"What's that?" I asked, nodding toward a stuffed ostrich on his bed.

"Oh, that? That's George." Turned out that George was a major player during hospital visits. I saw him many times after that. Then a silence hung between us. *All right, that's it. I got nothin'.* I felt like I should go. Maybe he was shy, or maybe he didn't want me in there. I thought it would be good for me to leave, expeditiously. Besides, he was probably in the isolation room for a reason. He might literally have a cootie. I had to be on the lookout for that stuff.

"Well, I gotta go," I said. Then I thought, *You moron! Why would you say that? Where exactly do you have to get to? What pressing appointments do you have to keep in here? Dummy.*

"OK. See ya around," he said quietly but cheerfully as I left the room and closed the door behind me. *He'll see me around?* I wondered. *Does that mean he wants to see me around, or is he just acknowledging the fact that we'll both be in the same area due to our communal fate?*

Linda

I didn't hate Dr. Stein, but she didn't seem to take people's emotions into consideration. She was very by the book. I always preferred Wolff. It became routine to have Wolff do everything, so if he wasn't available, she might substitute for him and it'd put me on my ear.

Taking a break from chemo was great. It was nice not to feel as though I'd been knocked flat on my back and someone was standing on my chest preventing me from getting back up again. I was surprised how fast my hair grew back, and crazily enough, it was coming in blond. My original hair color was a medium brown, straight with some under curl. When it grew back the first time, it came back black and pin curly, and as it grew out the pin curls became ringlets. Now, here I was coming in blonde and straight.

Seeing Dr. Stein for a month was no picnic, but it could've been a lot worse. Mostly, my problem was that I missed Dr. Wolff. He knew everything about me, and I didn't like being cared for by a "stranger." While we were seeing Dr. Stein, we rarely saw Dr. Wolff—not even in the hallways—and I wondered if he still liked us. I had a brief panic attack when the thought occurred that he might assign me to Dr. Stein permanently.

Toward the end of the month, I had to come in for a marrow biopsy. This allowed them to do two things: see if my marrow was healthy enough for harvesting yet, and check for cancer cells. I went to the clinic for my biopsy, and they put us in the big exam room—the one with the storage shelves in it. After Kaylee accessed my port, Dr. Stein moved the exam table to the center of the room, and I put a gown on and laid face down. Kaylee wrapped a blood pressure cuff around my arm and snapped an E.T. light on my finger. The little monitor near my head started squiggling with vital information. She was injecting stuff into the line, saying, "We're going to give you a little anesthetic. You'll be able to hear us and respond, but you won't care about much." It took ten minutes or so for it to start working; then I closed my eyes and dozed. The last thing I saw was Mom sitting in the chair by the door. Next thing I knew, I felt a dull pain on my back right hip. I tried to move away from it, but someone said to hold still. That seemed like a fine idea, so I did. Finally, the pain released and I started to doze again. Then, I felt it on my right side, and was more alert this time. This one hurt more. I started to move when Dr. Stein said,

"Just a little longer, OK? Lindsey, I need you to hold still…" Finally, the pain released, and I dipped back into my doze, punctuated occasionally by Kaylee asking me to take a big breath. When I woke up again, the first thing I saw was Mom sitting in the chair by the door.

"How'd it go?" I asked.

"Oh, I wasn't in here for it. Right after you went to sleep they shuffled me out to the waiting room," Mom said.

"Oh," I said. I hadn't heard the door open either time. I wasn't allowed to get up right away, so we waited in the exam room for a while. Dr. Wolff came in eventually.

"Dr. Stein said your marrow looked really good. It's nice and red. We'll be doing the harvest as soon as we can. When would be good for you?" As we were talking about scheduling, Dr. Norman popped in the door.

"How'd everything go?" he asked eagerly.

"It went really well. We'll do the harvest next week," Mom said.

"How does it work?" I asked. "Just like today?"

"Uh, no, not quite," Dr. Wolff said. "We'll be taking quite a lot of marrow. You're going to need three units of blood afterward. In order to get that much, we'll be using larger needles, so you'll have some small marks along your iliac crest."

"Let's just say you won't be wearing a bikini this summer!" Dr. Norman said cheerfully. Yeah, like I would anyway. Hello! Big scars across my abs *and* back! Not to mention the little one on my chest from the port.

During the car ride home, I was thinking about the operation. Should be pretty easy, compared to the others. I had almost no pain after this biopsy. I'd be under general anesthetic again, and I'd have to stay a night in the hospital. No sweat.

On the morning of my marrow harvest, we were at the hospital at seven a.m. Of course, I was abiding by the "no food for twelve hours before surgery" rule and was anxious to get this over with so I could eat. By now, this whole surgical thing was routine: lose the clothes (including the underwear this time), watch, jewelry, and nail polish. Then down to preop where they brief you on anesthesia—they didn't say much anymore; I told them I knew how it worked. Wheel into the operating room, scoot from the gurney to the table, get the gas mask, and good night.

Waking up, however, was definitely not routine.

I opened my eyes, as usual, to see a nurse standing over me, saying, "Lindsey can you hear me? If you can hear me, I need you to open your eyes. Can you wake up, Lindsey?"

I opened my eyes, looked at her, and registered what had happened before I started screaming in pain. I felt like my entire hip area had been torn apart.

"Are you in pain?" she asked dumbly. I continued screaming. It was all I was capable of. She pushed something in my port and I went back to sleep.

I was awoken again by Karen and the transportation guy. I was in my room—a double this time—and they wanted me to scoot from the gurney to my bed. I started whimpering because the pain was back.

Karen said, "Hey, girl! Can you scoot your little butt onto your bed for me?"

"It hurts…" I was doing my best to not cry.

"Don't worry. We'll take care of you, but I need you in your bed first. Do you want us to move you?"

"No!" I was awake for that one. God, if I felt bad now, I didn't want *anyone* moving me. Except Dr. Wolff. He could do it right, but he wasn't around. I thought for a second about the best way to move myself while keeping my hips straight. I thought if I could inch my legs, then my torso, then my legs, then my torso, I should be able to get comfortable in four movements or less. I started with my left leg, sliding it to my left and then went to move the right leg—but it wouldn't move! I stopped, shocked, and tried to wiggle my toes. Nothing. My right leg was paralyzed!

"I can't move my leg!" I said, highly alarmed.

"Do you want me to move it for you?" Karen asked.

"No!" I pleaded. Still trying to keep my hips as stationary as possible, I propped myself up on my elbows and nudged my right leg to the left with my hand. Inch by inch, I was able to shove myself over onto the bed, not without discomfort. After Dad tucked me all in, Karen came back with some Demerol and a bag of blood. She pushed the Demerol through my line as I looked at her skeptically.

"It won't work," I said. "It never does."

"It might," she said. I started feeling delightfully spacey and tired as I watched her hang the bag of blood on Stand-ley.

I awoke to Travis and Dad watching cartoons, which meant it was about four o'clock in the afternoon. I looked up at Stand-ley, who was decorated with a full bag of blood. Either I'd slept through the first transfusion, or I'd barely blinked. I slept again.

When I awoke again, it was dark out. I remembered my lame leg and tried to move it. Nothing. Not even a wiggle. Not even at my toes. Dr. Wolff came in after a while and told us that everything went very well, that the blood looked good, and everything went quickly.

"Dr. Wolff! I can't move my right leg!" I was afraid I'd never walk again.

"That was Dr. Stein's side," he said, as if relieved. "Can you feel this?" He pinched me on the foot.

"Yeah," I said.

"Don't worry. Sometimes those nerves can get pinched because we're working so hard."

Dad piped up. "How hard is it, to pull out the marrow?"

"It's a workout!" Dr. Wolff exclaimed, eyebrows raised. "You really get in there and you're pumping so hard you work up a sweat." I had a mental image of he and Dr. Stein, one on each side, holding giant needles and thrusting away at my hip bones, the syringes filling up with red. "We'll take a peek tomorrow, how's that?" he asked me. I nodded and he went home for the night.

Pretty soon, I had to pee. There was no catheter to bail me out this time. I buzzed the nurse. "Kar-ren! I gotta pee!"

"OK," she crackled. "I'll be in." She came in with a bedpan. I'd never used one of those before. She tucked it under me. I tried with all my might to pee, but I could not overcome a lifetime of training to *not* pee while in bed. I guess I didn't have to go *that* badly.

"Karen! I can't! Can I have the commode?" I'd gotten quite used to this little convenience. When you pee as much as I do in the hospital, it's nice to not have to walk all the way out to the bathroom in the middle of the night.

"You're not supposed to get up yet. Dr. Stein doesn't want those holes to pop open and bleed. We might not be able to stop it."

I was seriously uncomfortable now. "Kar-ren! Come on!"

"All right, I'll call her." She left and I waited, counting the seconds, willing my bladder muscles to constrict, *constrict*. After what seemed like a decade, she came back wheeling the commode. I rejoiced in all its glory.

"Just go slow, and be careful. And when you're done, it's back to bed with you. No bleeding!" I dragged my dead leg out of bed, slowly, mindful of my hips—but for once, the Demerol was working. Choirs sang Handel's "Alleluia!" while I peed. I'd never felt such pleasurable relief.

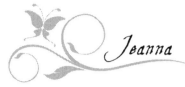

I got a phone call from Linda at work, and I instantly bailed, leaving my boss in the lurch. She was rushing Wes to the hospital and had left Lindsey and Travis at home. She told me, "I'm taking Wes to the hospital, but Lindsey has to go to the clinic today and Travis needs someone to watch him." Wes had had chest pains that morning and they were afraid it was a blood clot. Even Wes thought he was going to die that day.

So I ran over and picked up the kids, and we went to the clinic. Kaylee was working on Lindsey and asked, "Where's Linda?" I said carefully, "Well, she's taking Wes to the hospital because they think he has a blood clot." She kept her face perfectly calm and said conversationally, "Oh." We were trying to be calm and not alarm Lindsey or Travis (although he was well occupied with a toy tractor). The "clot" turned out to be anxiety attacks.

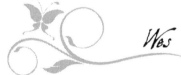

This was the winter from hell. One morning we all were walking through the double doors into 14A. I was on crutches and Lindsey was looking gray and sick. Travis had just had his surgery, too. Dr. Wolff saw us all from down the hall and gave us this look, shaking his head. That look said to me, "Jesus, what more does this family have to go through?"

While February was a good month for me, Dad was not faring nearly as well. Since the original accident, he'd had several surgeries. They managed to rebuild his leg with plates, pins, and screws, but the bone graft they'd placed in there died because he'd picked up a bug from the river water. They reopened him, cleaned it out, covered it with a skin graft, and he spent the next few months taking IV antibiotics at home. They gave him a double Hickman line, and he took vanco every day, just like I did when I had pneumonia. We kept it in the fridge, and I loathed the way it smelled. Keeping my bedroom door shut kept most of it out. In the end, they harvested a large amount of his marrow—they used some sort of scoop contraption instead of the needles they used on me—and transplanted it where his bone should be. Then, they took one side of his *abdominus rectus* muscle and transplanted it over the whole site. It was supposed to provide a blood supply and keep everything clean and healthy in there. It worked. Over my treatment protocol, he went from thigh-high casts to walking casts, and slept every night in the La-Z-Boy in the living room because he couldn't get to the bedroom in the basement. When they'd do skin grafts, they'd take them from his upper thighs, so he always had great big red patches on his legs that he said didn't hurt. I didn't believe him.

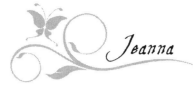

Jeanna

I went in to see Wes one day before a surgery and he just broke down. He was so alone. I ended up spending all day there. It reminded me that you really have to be there for people when they're sick. Our brother Roger and my husband Jeff came in the next morning and had a great visit. No one should go into surgery feeling as bad as Wes did.

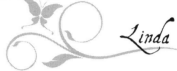

Linda

One of the cats scratched Travis, and he developed masses in three lymph nodes. I was totally freaked out that he had lymphoma. Dr. Wolff said, "No, it's not that. Don't worry about it." But we'd had enough stuff happen to us in recent years that was just so impossible that I decided to have them out to know for sure one way or the other. Because they weren't going down on their own.

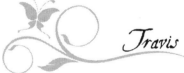

Travis

I had these pajamas that looked like a basketball jersey, and like a jersey, they were reversible. But they weren't sewn up all the way and looked a little like a kangaroo pouch. We had kittens at the house, so I'd put the kittens in the pouch and walk around with them. Eventually, one of them scratched me and the infection spread up my arm.

After the cat scratched me and the infection started to travel, we noticed a small lump in my armpit was getting bigger, and I thought to myself, What is that? That's kinda big. *It hurt to the touch. Then the fever came. Everyone got scared because my fever spiked to 107°F, and they took me to the emergency room. The doctors said they didn't know what was causing it and they wanted me to pee in a cup. I didn't want to and I told them that. "By the way, that's really weird," I added. Dad tried to help me pee in the cup, but it was a lost cause. Luckily, my fever started to go down on its own later, and they sent me home without peeing in any cups.*

Of course, I got to have a rad surgery with a scar and everything. Lindsey told me that everything is funny when you're on the laughing gas. So when I went to surgery I asked the doctors, "Is it true that everything is funny in here? Even bad jokes?" The doctors shrugged, probably thinking, Yeah, sure, kid. I don't know. I just work here. *But I was determined to find out. So after they gassed me I told them to start telling jokes. One of the doctors starts telling a story, "So awhile back, I hurt my nose because I ran into a wall." I started laughing uncontrollably. Then they made me count back from ten, and I was out.*

They decided not to sew my arm shut after the surgery so it could drain. The major benefit to this was that it looked like a mouth. I would make it "talk." While some people put lipstick on their hand to make a hand puppet, I used my armpit. But this also meant that they had to pack it full of gauze every day. I didn't mind at first. They said, "This might hurt a little." But then it hurt a lot. I mean, a lot. *It took six people to hold me down so they could stuff the incision with their nasty little tweezer-things. God, I hated that.*

So Dad and I were invalids together. Then Travis had his own bout in the hospital in December when Mom felt a large mass under his arm. She feared the worst: lymphoma. And considering all that had happened to our family in the last couple years, why *shouldn't* it be lymphoma? Turned out that he had Cat Scratch Fever. I remember when his diagnosis came down, and Mom said, "Cat scratch fever? Really? I thought that was just a Ted Nugent song." Apparently, one of the kittens on the farm—that we'd named Larry after Dr. Wolff—carried the virus, and Travis did something to the cat that earned him a scratch. Instead of the infection resolving itself, it seemed to bind up in his lymph nodes, and the mass just kept getting bigger.

By this time, Mom was the only one in the family left standing, and spent her days scrambling between hospitals and clinics making sure that we were all well taken care of. Travis's incision had been left open for drainage purposes, and it had to be packed periodically. This, needless to say, is not a *comfortable* experience.

It took almost every staff member in the clinic to hold him down and get it in there, while he kicked and fought and wailed protests. The other patients would peer out of their rooms in the direction of the screams, some with horrified looks on their faces. One little boy asked, "Is that kid in there getting a spinal tap? Ooh, I *hate* those."

I am unbelievably impressed with the staff at Doernbecher. That those doctors and nurses come to work every day and work on these little children. It seems to me that every new face they meet has a 50/50 chance of seeing Christmas that year. And they do a phenomenal job dealing with that every day. I remember a girl, about sixteen, who came in with leukemia. She was bawling in unbelievable pain. That girl did not live to see Christmas. I remember feeling guilty when we got to bring Lindsey home. Because we were bringing a healthy child home when so many other parents wouldn't get that. So in the end, I actually felt lucky. I think that statement will ring hollow and empty on most ears because it's probably something no one can understand unless they've walked in the shoes that the four of us walked in that year.

I resolved to myself if I ever had money to donate, if I ever became a wealthy man, the children's hospitals would get my money. It's a truly heartbreaking thing to go to these places and see the toddlers getting all the pokes and procedures and feeling sick every day. They can't possibly understand why Mommy and Daddy are putting them through all this pain.

If there is a silver lining in all of this, aside from the fact that Lindsey survived and became a strong person because of it, it was that she was old enough to have some understanding as to what was happening and why.

When I wasn't on 14A for one reason or another, or in the clinic with Dr. Wolff, I was more often than not at home. On the days I did go to school, I would sometimes only be able to pull a half day. Sometimes, toward the ends of my "breaks" right before I'd start a new cycle, I'd feel pretty good, and full days were fairly easy. Surprisingly, I received no taunting from the boys in my class, nor was I the butt of anyone's jokes—or not that I was aware of, anyway. People were curious about my routines, how I was feeling, and about that port. They always wanted to know about it. One boy said, "Oh, man, it would be cool to have that in the middle of my forehead." Ew.

My favorite thing to do was be around my horse. Because of the weakness, I'd handed over most of the exercise responsibilities to my cousin, Erin, who was hoping for a horse of her own someday. I simply wasn't able to get out there enough to ride, and good ol' Misty was getting flabbier and fatter every day. It was quite a departure from her previous sleek, shiny, and toned self. I could tell that the extra weight and sedentary lifestyle were affecting her feet—and she never really was sound to begin with.

Riding was a major release for me. It was the only part of my life where I didn't have to worry about inhaling some kind of virus or someone staring at me. It was a time that I could be pain-free, worry-free, and have quiet reflection. On days I was unable to ride, I enjoyed simply being in the barn because the smells were very comforting. The mixture of dirt, hay, horse sweat, and the sweet smell of leather were very normalizing. On bad days, I could go out there and groom Misty and feel better. She was a giant pet therapist. If I was feeling especially weak, for safety purposes I would double up with my cousin Erin, and it's a good thing we did, because it came in very handy.

It was an overcast day with rain misting down on us. Erin was with me, and we saddled up English style. I preferred English because it was more of a workout and, I felt, required more skill than Western. We had ridden down the pasture road to the hay field, where the ground was level and the grass was short. We decided to take turns, so Erin dismounted and I rode off, planning on working some patterns, just like we do at the shows. Misty was bad mannered, having spent most of the winter riderless, and was after the grass at her feet. I gave her a quick, "pay attention to me" spur and pushed her into a canter, doing figure eights. After a few loops, I felt she was performing a little better, and I relaxed my hands. She promptly planted her feet and bent her head down in the grass, and I promptly went right over it. I found myself on my butt in the grass in front of her, hearing her munching away behind me.

I checked myself to see if I'd broken or sprained anything. I hadn't. I checked for bleeding or bruising. There was none. The ground was soft that day. My ego was bruised, nonetheless. I hadn't been strong enough to stay on. It was the first time I'd ever fallen from a horse since I'd started riding four years before. I was stunned. Had the last part of my life that I controlled been stripped from me? I could feel the hot lump in my throat growing and hot tears stinging my eyes, threatening to burst over my cheeks. I looked at Misty, chowin' down on grass, and was suddenly very angry with her. Then, I was angry with myself for not being able to perform to my own expectations.

Erin came running up. "Are you OK?" she asked fervently.

"Yeah, I'm fine," I retorted, standing up. "Here," I thrust the braided leather reins into Erin's hands. "You ride. I can't do it, apparently." She threw the reins up over Misty's neck, stepped up into the saddle, and spurred her off. I sat down on the plow that sat on the edge of the hayfield and cried as I watched her put my horse through her paces with the ease and grace of any professional. It was official: I'd feared losing my control and strength from day one, and now it'd happened. Misty was such an important part of my childhood, and I felt as if she had been taken from me that day.

Karen shipped me off to the echo lab. Cyclophosphamide and doxorubicin have been known to cause heart issues, so they wanted to have a peek at mine. I liked the echo. No big deal. Painless, too. It was pretty interesting looking at all the valves flapping inside the heart, and see the different colors indicating blood flow. Wild.

The next day, Karen brought Fimo clay and a little toaster oven for me to make beads with. She had a box with little ones in it. Some of them were pretty detailed, with spirals and faces and all sorts of colors. I set about trying to mimic those beads and failed miserably. Mine came out of the oven looking like a big stupid lump instead of petite and perfectly cylindrical. But in the end, I had enough blue and purple beads to string a necklace for myself. Fimo became a favorite hospital past time and a crafty fad that year, but I never did manage to sculpt a little face.

Of course, following that cycle of chemo, I ended up back in the hospital again. This time I was in the room where I'd met Chris. I checked the board and couldn't find his name. That was too bad. I wanted a do-over. I wouldn't be such a dork this time. I realized with some dismay that I was the oldest patient on the ward that week by a good five years.

One afternoon, a few days into isolation, after my fever had been down for a day or so, I was sitting around (there's not much else to do in isolation) watching the Disney Channel. I decided to call Holly. Maybe she could come up tonight or tomorrow. Sometimes Wolff let us have sleepovers. Her brother, Devin, answered the phone. Now, Devin was the closest thing I had to a big brother. He was loud; he swore a lot, was equal parts totally obnoxious and inextricably cool. He did his duty as big brother and spent a fair amount of his time picking on Holly. He would always try to sit on her and fart. I never understood it, and I supposed I should be trying to help Holly, but the bottom line was that the whole thing was absurdly funny. He *was* actually pretty clever and managed to have us in stitches occasionally. Devin was generally very nice to me and would tell me to let him know "the second anyone caused any trouble" for me. Like he was going to go out and break their knee caps for it.

"Is Holly there?" I asked.

"No. This is Lindsey, isn't it?" he asked me.

"Yeah. I'm on Fourteen A and was hoping she could come up maybe tonight."

"You're in the hospital *again*? God." I could hear him chewing gum.

"Yeah," I scoffed.

"Hey, I got some books that you might like to read. Holly can bring them to you," he said, offhandedly.

I made a face. Since when did *Devin* like to read books? "Oh yeah? What are they?" I asked.

"I've got two here. The first one is called, *Under the Grandstands* by Seymore Buttz..." There was expectant silence on the line. At first I didn't realize that he'd delivered a punch line. Then it hit me. Seymore Buttz. See more butts. *Under the Grandstands* by Seemore Butts. It was hilarious! I started giggling, and he continued,

"...and the other is *The Yellow River* by I.P. Freely." I was cracking up by this time. He talked to me for a few more minutes before saying he'd tell Holly I called and hanging up. I sat propped up in bed smiling as I laughed to myself about I.P. Freely.

I was in the clinic one day for dehydration and nausea. Dr. Wolff decided I would stay for the day and get IV fluids. Kaylee accessed me and plugged me in to the saline drip, and I walked into the day room, where there was an empty bed. Mom followed with the omniscient Louis Vuitton bag full of books, magazines, water bottles, and a box of Chicken in a Biskit. I laid down and looked over at the other bed. It was empty, but there was a woman sitting in the chair next to it, reading. After a few minutes, a tall young man came walking through the door, pushing his Pole-ish friend on which an enormous bag of bright yellow liquid hung. Chris.

"Oh, hello," he said to me in his usual quiet but cheerful manner as he settled himself on the other bed.

"Hi!" I said, smiling. *Try to not be so much of a dweeb this time, Lindsey.*

Patsy was fixing some Benadryl in the IV drip. "You two know each other?" she asked me.

"Yeah, Karen introduced us," I said.

"That's nice," Patsy said. "You two are just about the oldest patients we have. You probably have quite a bit in common." She winked at me and smiled. What did that mean?

Kaylee pushed the Super Nintendo cart into the day room and left. Patsy said, "Hey, you guys into the Nintendo?"

"Sure, I'll play," Chris said. Patsy gave us each a controller, and we occupied ourselves with *Super Mario World* while Mom and Chris's mom talked. Her name was Sue, and they lived in Eugene. I thought that was pretty far to have to drive in and see the doctor. Chris was the oldest of three kids. Chris sometimes had to come up for treatment alone and stay at the Ronald McDonald House because they lived so far away. I felt sad for him that he couldn't always just go home after his treatments like I could, but Sue was there with him as often as she could be.

They talked and talked, and Chris and I played on, but before the Benadryl started working, I got that special feeling that said it was time to throw up. I paused the game, put my controller down, grabbed the green plastic tub, and spewed away, delighting, as always, in the unique bouquet of stomach acid. Mmm, boy. When I was finished, I looked up and saw that Chris was in the middle of throwing up, too. His mom sat next to him with an arm on his shoulders and a paper towel at the ready.

As Patsy came in to fetch my vomit, my Mom gestured to Chris, saying, "I hope we didn't cause that." I shot a dirty look at her, thinking, *Oh, you're sorry I caused his barf? What about my barf?* Sue shrugged and said softly, "Oh, no, not at all. We throw up about this time every day." Chris finished, wiped his mouth with the paper towel, sighed, and fell back again on the bed. Sue took the bucket and handed it off to Patsy who'd returned after rinsing mine out. Chris looked exhausted, and I can't say that I felt that sprightly myself. The Benadryl was taking hold, and my muscles were all starting to twitch as they relaxed. Within fifteen minutes I think we were both asleep.

The next cycle of chemo I received brought with it some unsolicited and very unwanted drama.

About halfway through the week, I was ordered to go through a battery of tests. Firstly, I went to Audiology. Some of the drugs I'd received were known to cause hearing issues. Not deafness, but ringing in the ears (tinnitus) is a known side effect, and my ears had been ringing off the hook for quite a while. When they wheeled me out of the South Hospital and to the Physician's Pavilion where Audiology was located, I started to get nervous. What if I was going to lose my hearing someday? No one had told me whether or not the ringing would end after treatment or whether or not it would get progressively worse. The transportation guy left me in my wheelchair in the hallway, and I waited for what seemed like hours. Finally, a man came out to get me, wheeled me into a little cubicle that was lined completely with what looked like charcoal gray egg-crate foam, and I moved from the wheelchair to the chair in the booth. He explained how it would work and then took my wheelchair with him in the hallway and closed the door behind him. I felt pressure on my ears when the door latched—the room must be very tight. After he was gone, it was absolutely, completely silent in there. Every breath, sniff, creak of the chair, and even blink were stark and almost deafening in comparison.

I was sitting at a counter. On it was a pair of headphones, with a telephone cord coming out of one side that plugged into a jack in the wall under the counter. In front of me was a large, plate-glass window. On the other side was an identical booth, also lined with the same charcoal gray egg crate. There was another pair of headphones on the counter and some equipment on which little lights of different colors blinked continuously. There was a little microphone. After a while, the man appeared on the other side of the glass and started shuffling some papers around and clicking on the equipment.

I heard nothing.

He picked up the earphones and motioned for me to do the same. I put them on and heard his voice.

"OK, so all we're going to do is play some tones in your headset, on each side of your head independently, and we'll see how much you can hear. When you hear the tone, raise your hand. Ready?" It sounded simple enough. I nodded.

"OK, give me a few seconds to start everything up in here." I waited. As I did, I started thinking. *What if I can't hear the tones? Should I pretend to hear the tones?* Oh, God, would I have to go through the rest of my life with a hearing aid? That would suck. In the headset I heard, "Here we go. Get ready." Oh boy, I was. My arm was tense, my hand at the ready. I listened hard. After a while, I heard the tiniest, high-pitched tone in my right ear—like the tone they play on the Emergency Broadcast System.

My hand shot up.

He would change the pitch of the tone, the ear he played it in, and the volume, and any time I heard it, my hand shot up. After a while, I felt like I was listening so hard that I wasn't sure if I was hearing the tone or not. I'd totally psyched myself out. Was I making it up? What if I raised my hand and he *wasn't* actually playing the tone? *Just chill out*, I told myself. *Relax. If you quit thinking about it so hard, you'll do better.* Finally, he spoke in the microphone again.

"OK, Lindsey, you can take your headset off and leave the room. We're finished. Go wait in the wheelchair, and I'll call transport for you. I'll have your results to take back to your doctor, too."

I waited another eternity for transportation. Why couldn't I just wheel myself? Eventually, I saw the telltale green jacket dodging between other patients in the office, coming toward me. Just as he got to me, the audio guy came up with a folder.

"Here you go," he said, smiling. Why was he smiling? Did I pass? Was he laughing at me because I failed? I wondered if I was allowed to open the envelope and read the reports—or if I'd even understand them.

Transportation brought me back to the ward and started to wheel me to my room, when Karen stopped him, saying I was scheduled for a GFR down in Nuclear Medicine. Off we went. I desperately hoped Nuclear Medicine had been remodeled since last I saw it. I wasn't interested in hanging out in Canary Yellow Hell for the next few hours.

When we got there, they took me right in. The isotope was warm and waiting. The nurse came at me with a butterfly tray. I yanked my arms in closer to my body. "Whoa there," I said, alarmed. "What are you doing? I've got a port."

"Do you want us to put it in your port? If we do we can't draw from your port because there'll be residue in there." I thought for a second. One butterfly to inject, or three butterflies to draw for the next hour and a half. I opted for the lesser of the two evils. Not that it was any easier. They fought with my veins for ten minutes before they were able to get in. I was a wreck. Watching them inject the isotope didn't help. The idea that everyone was OK with injecting radioactive isotopes into me was highly bothersome. After they were done and they'd given the butterfly a good flush, transportation came back to get me and bring me to 14A.

After the first hour, Karen came in with a butterfly tray.

"No, Karen! You can draw from my port! They used a butterfly to inject it."

"Oh, good." She disconnected me from the drip and screwed a syringe on the end of my port tube. She pulled the blood, flushed the line, and plugged me back into the drip. Thirty minutes later she came back and did the same. Finally, another thirty minutes later she came back for the last one. My parents had shown up during the blood draw hour and waited with me.

After a while, Dr. Wolff appeared, and pointed a finger at me. "You been to CT yet?" he asked.

"No," I said frowning, "I didn't know I was supposed to go." He seemed to sigh heavily, and then abruptly spun around and left. He came back after a few minutes saying, "They're going to get you in this afternoon. Transport will be coming for you."

"Why am I getting a CT?" I asked, slightly worried.

"It's time," he answered. "It's been awhile." Sure enough, transport showed up again, and this time the wheelchair took me to the eleventh floor. Diagnostic Imaging.

CAT scans always seem to take forever. By the time I was actually on the table and sliding into the giant donut, I was feeling hungry. *Oh, what I wouldn't give for a box of Froot Loops right now,* I thought. My parents were behind the wall in the booth with the technicians, watching. They slid me through to my mid chest.

"OK, you know the routine. I'll tell you when to breath and when to hold. Let's get this done, yeah? It's getting late." The donut whirred and clicked and buzzed. I breathed, held, breathed, held, breathed, held, and breathed again until the speaker told me to stop. Then I waited, freezing. Mom came in and got me a blanket fresh out of the warmer. It reeked of antibacterial cleanser, but it was warm. Eventually, the tech came in, said I could dress, and we headed back to 14A. When we got there, Dr. Wolff was at the nurse's desk, and Mom went to talk to him. I headed for my room that was in view of the nurse's station, and turned around. I was watching them talk, feeling glad that the day was over, when Denise came up and tried to guide me in the room. Just as I started to turn in, I saw Dr. Wolff say something to Mom, and she buried her face in her hands and started to cry. "Oh, God, not again!" He gestured for them to come with him to a private room where they could talk.

It was back.

"What's happening? What's wrong?" I demanded as I started to move forward. Denise stopped me, and she and another nurse gently but strongly pulled me into the room. I was shrieking.

"What happened? What's wrong with the films? What did they see? *Tell me what they see!*" Denise was trying to block my view of the hallway—an impossible task considering her spindly build—and talking to me quietly. The other one said, "I'm going to call Child Life," and she left the room. I would not be mollified. I couldn't see Dr. Wolff or either of my parents in the hall anymore. I started to cry. *Not again*, I thought. *I can't do this anymore.* Why *won't they tell me what happened?* I heard Denise's voice saying something about staying calm until we heard from Dr. Wolff. *Screw that*, I thought. *I saw what happened out there.*

I was suddenly very angry.

I hated being a minor. You always found things out last. And people always treated you as a child, regardless of your ability to grasp what was going on. Did they forget that I was practically an adult? I mean, really, think about what had happened in the last year and a half. It wasn't happening to Dr. Wolff, or Mom or Dad or any other adult. It was happening to *me*, in *my* body and I *still* was the last person to know anything. I was angry at everyone. It didn't matter who, or whether they were even related to what was going on right now. The only one I wasn't angry with was God–I didn't think He actually had a direct hand in what was happening to me. But I know plenty of people who would've been angry with God right from the start.

Denise had finished with my IV and was simply waiting in the room with me while I seethed silently and dripped tears all over the place. Where *were* they? What was taking so long? Were they going over which painful procedures I hadn't had yet and now was eligible for? Were they planning any funerals in there? Which organ would I lose next? Would they use the marrow they took out? Thousands of possibilities flooded my mind. Perhaps I'd just be on chemo for the rest of my life.

Someone knocked on the door. Denise opened it. It was the woman from Child Life. What was her name? Colleen, that's right. I'd seen her wandering the halls. She was a small woman, both thin and short. She was maybe in her late forties or early fifties. I couldn't tell for sure. Her hair was short, thick, and curly. Like Carla's on *Cheers*. She had a bunch of paper and crayons in her hands. "Hi, Lindsey," she said. "I'm Colleen."

I stared at her openmouthed. They had sent someone to *color* with me? I wanted desperately to say, "Look, lady, I got bigger things to worry about here. I don't have time to color with you.

Get the hell out." Of course, I wasn't raised to say whatever graced my brain. Few people are.

"Heard you had a bad day," she said. She sat down in the chair next to my bed. "It sounds like you've been all over the place today, having some nasty things done." She was right about that. Audiology had freaked me out. Nuclear Medicine was no picnic, by far, and finally this CAT scan was the icing on the cake.

"You know, sometimes when we're angry or sad, it helps to express it physically," she said. "One safe way to do that is with art. You can scribble hard and furiously, and it helps you get out what you're feeling." I stared at her. She put three or four large pieces of construction paper on my bed table, and handed me a box of crayons. I picked up a crayon and looked at the paper for a moment, not knowing what to draw. I saw her pick up a crayon and scribble black lunatic corkscrews all over her piece of paper. I set the crayon to the paper and scribbled. Hard. I broke a few crayons, and when I was done scribbling, I tore all the paper up and threw it. It went everywhere. I stopped, feeling a light sweat, and suddenly feeling guilty for acting out and making such a mess. I wasn't used to behaving that way, and I was embarrassed.

Colleen wasn't. She smiled at me. "Feels pretty good, doesn't it?"

I looked at her and realized she was right. I heaved a cleansing sigh and nodded. I did feel better. I felt calmer and clearheaded now. I wasn't completely unwound, but at least my horns and forked tail had disappeared for the moment. Now I was just anxious.

Dr. Wolff and my parents came in after a long while. I waited expectantly, looking at them all in turn. It was Dr. Wolff who spoke. "Your scan had something interesting on it." Interesting. Interesting? What the hell did that mean? Dr. Wolff was not the type to beat around the bush. "There is a spot. It's right near where the incision was made, and it's slightly odd-looking. We thought at first that it was a new tumor, but now I don't think it is." I sighed heavily. He continued, "It appears to be scar tissue. It's denser than your normal tissue, so it shows up in the scan. We'll do another scan later, and that will tell us for sure whether it has changed at all, but it sure looks to me like scar tissue." Scar tissue! Ew. We'd all made all this fuss over a *scab*?

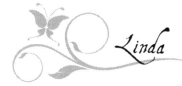

Linda

By the second round of treatment, you start to adjust and think, OK, this is just how it's got to be now. *But I don't think I ever felt like this process became "normal." I never even felt comfortable when we finished that first protocol of chemo and radiation. It wasn't until after the relapse was treated that I felt, "OK, we got this."*

The executive decision was made, about midway through May, that I'd had enough. And I agreed. I'd gotten a little stir crazy over the past couple months, being in and out of the hospital so much and with that whole scar tissue scare. The last time I'd ended up with a fever and Dr. Wolff ordered me to 14A, I caught myself rocking back and forth on my bed anticipating another trip to isolation. I looked like one of those crazy people you see in movies, and that scared me. I didn't want to go crazy on top of the whole cancer thing.

Knowing that I was on the cusp of being done changed my outlook entirely. I was only a month from graduation day, my hair would be coming back soon, and I was excited to get out of Forest Grove and (hopefully) go to high school in Portland. I was looking forward to a summer with my horse, and maybe making a Wish.

PART TWO:

The After Math

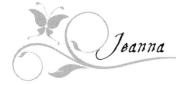

Jeanna

I can look at myself, at my age, and be thankful that I can still do the things I like to do, and that I'm still here and able to do all that I want to do. I know it's just a phone call away, or a lump away or a sudden bleed away. We have to appreciate it right now because it can all change in a flash. It's never subtle. It's like getting hit by a truck.

I'd learned about Make-A-Wish earlier in the winter, and seeing that Misty was getting so old and my skills were outgrowing her, I, of course, wanted a new horse. Incidentally, I went with Sharon one day to the barn where she boarded and trained her show horse, Buddy. There was a black mare also living there, and she was for sale. Her name was "Intimidating Dollie." I loved her the second I saw her shiny black coat. She was petite—only about 14:2 hands tall (about fifty-six inches at the withers), with skinny legs and tiny hooves to match. She had two little white anklets on her back legs. The trainers let me ride her while Sharon was working with her horse. She had an odd side-to-side jog, but I clicked with her instantly. It was a pleasure riding a horse that had been broken and trained with the purpose of showing in mind. She understood commands for lead changes and executed patterns with a minimum of effort on my part. Best of all, I had no anxiety about getting pitched off the front. She wasn't going to screech to a sudden halt and dip down for a mouthful of grass. I loved her instantly. I wanted to Wish for her.

Two Make-A-Wish Foundation volunteers came out to the house to meet me and take my request. I told them all about Dollie. She was perfect. When I was done with my breathless description, I waited for them to tell me they'd go get her. They didn't say that. They did say that I had to come up with a "Plan B Wish" in case they couldn't get Dollie for me. It hadn't occurred to me that they might not be able to make this wish come true. With clenched teeth and more than a little embarrassment I remembered that Dollie came with a five-thousand-dollar price tag. That was a lot of money.

"I'm going to have to think about that," I said. That night as I lay in bed, I thought more about it. I wanted Dollie so desperately, that I couldn't imagine her not being a part of my life. She was what I'd wanted for years. A real show horse. A well-trained horse. We could be so successful...I'd surely qualify for State on her, perhaps go all the way to the Oregon Quarter Horse circuit. Dare I think it, even the World Championships? The very idea dazed me. Popping the dreamy image of us standing in front of the World Championships sign, Dollie's neck draped in flowers and me wearing a shiny new buckle, I brought myself back from idealisms. How could I make this work? Could I wish for something more expensive so that they'd have to get Dollie? I immediately felt guilty for thinking about taking advantage of Make-A-Wish like that. They'd probably just say no. But what else did I want *that badly*? I knew a lot of kids wished for Disneyland. But we'd already been there once. Some kids wanted their families to go on a big tropical vacation, but I didn't care about sunning myself in the Caribbean. What did I love? That horse. OK, what else?

And then a solution came to my mind. It'd likely be more expensive, but it wouldn't be contrived. There were two things that had helped me through the last six months: my friends, and *The Late Show with David Letterman*. Dave had kept me company at 11:35 p.m. each night in the hospital and got me laughing before I fell asleep. I adored that show. Sometimes I made Karen stay and watch it with me, just to the Top Ten List. What if I could wish to see David Letterman? To meet him, or be on the show? Of course, I wanted my family with me, but I also wanted my friends to be there—Holly and some of the other girls from school, and maybe my cousins. That was it! That would be the ultimate! New York City! To meet David Letterman! And maybe be on the show. I was set. One wish would mean happiness for years, and the other would be the coolest week of all time. We submitted my Plan B Wish and sat back to wait.

I finished my treatment in May and had one last bout with pneumonia before it was all over. The day I walked out of Doernbecher was the most liberating day of my life. I didn't care what happened in the future, I was just glad that this part was over.

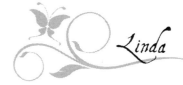

Health insurance was an absolute nightmare. I didn't want to have to be too concerned with that, because my job was to take care of Lindsey. So I gave it all up to Wes to take care of. It was incredibly hard to pay off the medical bills, especially with Wes down from an injury for almost a year. I could only work part time in order to take care of everyone. I don't even know how we did it.

On my next trip to see Dr. Wolff, after my exam, I saw Chris and his mom in the day room. He was under a couple blankets, attached to the biggest bag of electric-yellow fluid I had ever seen. "What's going on?" I asked, smiling, as I peered around the corner into the room. It cheered me to see him. They explained that he was getting some serious doses of antifungals because he had some sort of stubborn infection. Apparently, if it didn't work, he would have to go to some other hospital to get another treatment that would. I figured that meant going across the river to Emmanuel hospital. I felt a moment of cursory worry over him, and then it was gone.

After graduation, and just before June, I had another trip to the clinic. Wolff wanted one last peek before I headed off on my senior trip. I asked about Chris while I was in there, and someone mentioned that he was in Bethesda, Maryland, for some sort of experimental treatment to eradicate that infection. I couldn't believe he still had it. I'd never had any kind of infection that took more than a week to rectify. I mean, when they're pounding you with antibiotics that are a mere shadow below the intensity of chemotherapy, you'd think that would kill anything. He had to be there for a couple months. Yuck. I couldn't imagine spending a couple months in the hospital. Bethesda. Where was that, anyway?

"Oh, hey, Maryland," Mom said, "That's right near where you'll be."

"It is?" I asked.

"Yeah, it's a suburb of DC."

"Maybe I could stop in and see him," I wondered aloud. Mom assured me that it was unlikely since I was part of a scheduled tour. Disappointed, I said, "Well, I'll write him letters and call him, then."

After the appointment, Mom and I decided to go up to 14A and say hi to the nurses up there. Then I remembered: how would I contact Chris if I didn't have an address or anything? Denise was on the floor that afternoon. "Denise, do you know where Chris is?" I asked.

"Chris Mason? Oh, he's such a nice boy, isn't he? He's in Maryland right now, I think," she said while scribbling notes in a file.

"Is there, like, an address or something? I want to send him some letters. It sounds like he'll be there for a long time."

She looked over at me. "Lindsey, that's so sweet of you!" She picked up the phone. "I'm going to call the medical center for you and get it." She put her pen down and went behind the desk. I waited while she was on the phone. After a few minutes, she took down some information on a piece of paper and handed it over to me, saying, "This is great that you want to write to him. He's just the nicest boy. He's so polite. And isn't he just the cutest?" She winked at me. I laughed back. Ha! Yeah...cute.

"What are we talking about here?" a voice behind me asked. I recognized it as Dr. Stein's. Denise said, "Lindsey is going to write to Chris Mason while he's cooped up in Bethesda. Isn't that nice?"

"Oh, *really?*" Dr. Stein cooed as she gave me the eye. "Well, woo-hoo!" There was something different about how she made the same basic comment that Denise did, and it irritated me. I knew what she meant; I wanted to yell out, "It's not like that! We're just friends!" I folded up the paper with the address on it, stuck it in my pocket, and we left for home.

"Dr. Stein made way too big a deal out of that," I snorted.

"Yeah, she did," Mom agreed.

The first week of June, I joined my class at the Portland International Airport where we boarded a DC-10 bound for Virginia. It was the biggest plane I'd ever seen. When my family and I were standing at the gate, waiting to board, I thought I recognized a face out of the corner of my eye. As I looked over at him, he looked at me. "Well, look. Lindsey VanDyke. How are ya?" It was Dr. Henricks—my surgeon.

"Dr. Henricks?" I asked. A small part of me silently wished Dr. Rainieri was with him. My parents looked over. "Dr. Henricks?" Mom exclaimed. "Wow, how funny that we run into you here! What are the odds?" She talked to him while we waited. He was there to pick up one of his kids from study-abroad in Europe. Mom told him all about my trip to Washington, DC. He beamed.

"You done with treatment now?" he asked.

"Yeah," I answered. "I finished a few weeks ago."

"You're looking good. Getting some color back, and it's always nice to see kids maintain their weight. That Zofran is a miracle." Maintain my weight, my butt. I'd *gained* about ten pounds since treatment started, and now my clothes were tight. The door opened to the gate he was waiting for, and people began filing out. He said good-bye and went up to find his daughter. Not long after, they called my gate. Mom handed me a huge bag full of different foods and snacks, and a dozen disposable cameras.

"Make sure you eat every few hours. I don't want you getting sick from low blood sugar. Here's lots of water for you, too." She looked me square in the eye. "*Do not* get dehydrated, there's no place for you to get IV fluids. Oh, and always, *always* wear sunscreen; your skin is very sensitive still…"

"Yeah, I know, Mom."

"And there's a wheelchair on the bus for you, just in case, so if you feel too tired to keep up, *use it.*" No way.

"Yeah OK, Mom."

"Be safe. Stay in groups. Don't go off by yourself anywhere. Watch out for weirdoes…"

"*OK,* Mom!" I was getting agitated. I knew she'd recruited some of the other moms to supervise my food and fluid schedules and watch over me like a hawk. It's not like I was going by myself, after all. I hugged her and went over to Dad. He gave me a hug and said, "Be good kid, Bambino." His advice was always the same. I started to walk toward the gate to join Holly and a group of girls.

"Oh, Booie!"

I spun on my heel. "*What?* Mom!"

"We love you!" She was waving fanatically. As I handed over my boarding pass and entered the jetway, I heard Travis yammering, "Why does *Lindsey* get to go on the plane? *I* want to go on the plane! Lindsey gets to do *everything*." Yeah. Including cancer.

It was my first trip in a plane. I was amazed at how wide it was, with three columns of seats, two against the windows, five in the middle, and two more against the other windows. Yet, I was surprised at how small it felt, too. The ceilings weren't much higher than any of our heads.

Although my counts were high enough to travel, I still had some issues with food—especially if my blood sugar bottomed out. It wasn't pretty. I'd get angry and weepy and refuse to eat, which after a while would start the chain reaction vomiting. But that's what Mom's recruited chaperones were watching for. It got annoying.

Flying on a plane was so exciting. It was great to travel with all my friends. I wondered if Make-A-Wish was working on the New York trip—if it would be this much fun, I'd happily sacrifice the horse wish. After our stop in Chicago, I broke out my stationary and the address to the medical center in Bethesda. As I wrote, I thought about Chris and how much I enjoyed meeting him and his mom during treatment. It had become one of the highlights of this protocol. He was the only friend my own age I'd really made at the hospital since I was diagnosed. I admired him because it seemed like his situation was so much worse than mine, and he seemed to bear it quietly and without protest (unlike me, who protested constantly). He admired me because I took G-CSF shots every day (obviously he didn't know how ungracefully I did it). Denise had a point. He was the sweetest boy I'd ever met. He was very polite. And maybe...he was kind of cute. Maybe. For a boy, anyway. I wrote him a letter asking how he was, how the hospital there compared to Doernbecher, and detailing the finer points of my first trip on a jet.

When we walked out of the airport in Virginia, it was stifling. I'd never felt heat and humidity like that. It felt hard to breathe. I quickly learned that one week of hardcore tourism on the East Coast in early summer was almost more exhausting than six months of being in the hospital.

During the week, we saw Mt. Vernon, Jamestown, Yorktown, the Washington Monument, the Lincoln Memorial, the White House, the Jefferson Memorial, the Smithsonian museums of American and natural history, the National Holocaust Memorial Museum, and the Vietnam Memorial. We went to the U.S. Capitol Building—which is in no way easily accessed by wheelchairs, and where the security guards felt sorry for me and let me in the restricted gallery where I saw a lot of men in blue suits filibustering away. It was kind of boring, but everyone else was so excited about it that I didn't say so. We saw the Supreme Court, the Federal Reserve, Union Station, and Arlington Cemetery.

The most memorable moment I had, unrelated to the exhibits and tour of Washington, DC, occurred at Busch Gardens, when I had succumbed to the uncomfortable wheelchair. My coterie was arguing amongst themselves about who got to push me around—it didn't have big wheels, so I couldn't push myself. While they squabbled, two young men approached me. One was probably in his mid-twenties. He knelt down in front of my chair and said, "Hey, what type of cancer do you have?" A bit disconcerted by this overt and forward greeting, I wondered if this man was one of the "weirdoes" Mom told me to watch out for.

"I have Wilms Tumor. Kidney cancer," I mumbled.

"I had leukemia!" he exclaimed. "I just got done with treatment a few months ago!" I warmed up to him immediately. This was a kindred spirit. "Where are you going?" he asked us. We all looked at each other.

"How about that way?" one girl suggested, pointing to our left.

"Would you mind if I pushed your wheelchair?" the stranger asked. No one argued with him. We set off, this guy piloting my chair, his buddy walking beside him, and my friends traveling in a pack on either side of me. He said his name was Roger, and he asked me questions about my treatment and how I was doing these days. As he pushed me over the uneven pavement, the chair rattled and bumped and I thought, *How awful would it be to be stuck in one of these every day?* I asked him about which type of leukemia he had, mentioning that I had a friend who has AML. He said he'd had leukemia twice. We talked comfortably in cancer/hospital lingo that we'd both picked up. How many transfusions had I had? Had he ever taken Zofran? Where were we treated? And so on. Suddenly, I remembered: I had had cancer twice, too. I said, "Hey, me too! This was my second protocol."

"Really?" he asked, surprised. "Oh, it's an amazing experience, isn't it? Not fun, but still amazing." I had never thought of it that way. I had learned a lot about myself, and definitely about the human body—equal parts totally gross and totally rad. I'd met quite a few people who were now very important to me. *He's right*, I thought, *it was pretty amazing*. We stopped in front of a giant roller coaster.

"Hey, I've gotta go," he said. "But it was incredible to talk with you. Keep it up. Everything will turn out right in the end. Cancer is a horrible thing, but I just know that God is teaching us something through it." He and his buddy walked off in the direction we'd just come from. It felt pretty special meeting someone who knew exactly what I'd felt. Except for the God part. I thought that going through two cancers was a pretty crummy way to *learn* something. If God wanted me to learn something, he could've just *told* me.

By the time we were at Dulles a week later, I was definitely ready to return to the Pacific Northwest. I'd managed to not get lost, sunburned, or dehydrated—another girl did, though, and she was seriously *sick* all week and wouldn't listen to any of my antinausea suggestions. But the East Coast was for chumps. I couldn't understand why these people liked to live in all this heat and humidity. Especially back in George Washington times–they all wore so many layers of clothes! How could they survive here without air conditioning? I wanted to go home where the weather was mild and comfortable.

When I returned, I noticed a change in Misty. She was having an exceptionally hard time walking, and her limps were overtly obvious. Who could blame her? She'd been lame for most of her life, and she was pushing twenty-four. Despite my best efforts at soaking her feet and giving her big doses of Bute—a painkiller—she continued to get worse. Finally, at the end of the month, Dad decided the best thing we could do was put her down.

"You're not going to shoot her in the head, are you?" I asked, almost crying. On a farm, where things always needed to be economical and there was often a need for quick resolution to serious problems in livestock such as broken bones or births gone wrong, the shotgun could prove to be a quick and useful solution.

"No, I'm not gonna shoot her," he said, softly.

"So, I should call the vet?" I asked, and then I thought, *Where do you bury an 1100-pound horse?* "Wait, what will we do with her?"

"I don't know. I'll find out." Dad made some calls and found an organization that will pick up your horse, transport it somewhere in western Washington, euthanize it, and bury it. The next day, he came to me and said, "You should go say good-bye to Misty. I found some people who will take care of her and they're coming to pick her up at four a.m. tomorrow." So I went to her large indoor pen with some treats from the feed store that she always loved. I let her eat right out of the bag, as much as she wanted while I told her how great it was to have had her the last four years. She'd been a good horse. It really wasn't her fault I fell off that day, and I learned so much from her. When I'd said all I could, I dropped her some hay, locked the gate, and closed up the barn.

The next day I returned, wondering if she'd actually be gone. She was.

I thought about her that day, and whether or not she'd been put to sleep yet. I wondered how painful it was for her to stand in a trailer from here all the way to Washington. I wondered if she was scared, or if she was comfortable because she'd be around a bunch of other horses.

Now that there was no horse in my life at all, I was suddenly nervous about my Make-A-Wish. Before, I'd hoped more for the horse than for the New York trip, but now I was desperate. Horses were such a huge part of my life. It was the only sport I was even remotely good at, and it provided a lot of stress relief and quiet time. If Make-A-Wish granted me Dollie, I would definitely make the most of it. I would go as far as there is to go in 4-H, and I'd arrange it to have a shot at the Oregon Quarter Horse circuit, and maybe the World Championships, if I were good enough. My imagination ran off with me.

Just chill out. Try to take one step at a time.

A few days later, while Mom was putting the finishing touches for the big Fourth of July BBQ she was putting together, Make-A-Wish called. I was listening in the other room, trying to be cool but sweating with apprehension, and when she came in, I looked at her expectantly. "Well?" I demanded. She looked long at me.

"They weren't able to get Dollie for you. Someone already bought her." I heaved a sigh, brimming with disappointment and shattered brief hopes. It was fine. She was probably too expensive anyway. "And there's another thing," she continued, "they checked into the *Late Show*, and there is a minimum age of sixteen required to be in the audience." OK, so no horse *and* no *Late Show*. Damn.

"So what does that mean? There's just no wish?" I asked, incredulous. Now I was very disappointed. Everyone had built this up so big for nothing. They'd all gotten my hopes up about this Make-A-Wish thing, and I wasn't even going to get one? I felt crushed. I'd been on the cusp of getting the greatest gift anyone could get, and wham! Gone.

"No, they still want to talk to you about wishes, but we'll have to start over again." She watched me, as I sat looking at the floor, thinking. What else could I want? Nothing. I didn't want anything. No wish. Mom piped up, "Maybe we could go to Disneyland or something?"

"We've been there already," I said darkly.

"Well, what about Hawaii then? Or maybe Europe?" she posited. No, no. I didn't want to travel...I might just drop the whole thing. It would be stupid to wish for something simply for the sake of eking *something* out of them. I abandoned it and decided to take a walk to fantasize about how great it all *could* have been.

I ended up in the barn, where I overturned a five-gallon bucket and sat down, taking in the smells. A white cat with big tabby spots slithered down from the rafters to walk along the tops of the stall walls. She came toward me and jumped in my lap. She just sat there, flicking her tail, her motor purring. The sound was not unlike the pumps that were once connected to a certain pair of chest tubes I remembered all too well. I scratched behind the cat's ears, and as she blissfully drooled all over my jeans, I looked about the barn. The bridles hung on the wall, their bits glinting in the late sun. The saddle sat on a sawhorse, the pads and blankets on top, horsey side up to air out the sweat, of course. A partially eaten bale of hay lay at the end of the aisle, waiting to be fed for dinner that wouldn't come. The medical kit sat on a shelf, filled with Epsom salt, bandages, rolls of cotton, syringes, worming paste, hydrogen peroxide, and Bute—the equine equivalent to Toradol. The grooming bucket was near my feet filled with currycombs, hoof picks, brushes, mane conditioner, and fly spray. Misty's old fly mask was on the nail in front of the stall. Her telltale blue halter and red lead were gone. I put my face in my hands and cried while the cat serpentined around my ankles.

The Fourth of July dawned bright and hot. There were long tables borrowed from the church set up in our vast front yard with red, white, or blue vinyl tablecloths on them. Mom had put up flags everywhere. She filled up a huge blue plastic utility tub with ice and threw in a bunch of pop. They set up the barbeque. One of my uncles showed up with a couple of kegs.

I decided to wear black that day in a vain effort to mask the extra ten pounds I'd gained on chemo. And because I was mourning. My hair still wasn't growing, which I found disconcerting, so I topped my head with a black derby. I put on the eyeliner that Mom liked me to wear to pretend that I had lashes. By noon, people started showing up. Mom had invited at least a hundred people: friends, relatives, acquaintances, clients, etc. By midafternoon, the party was going strong. Our place was thronged with people. I was showing a bunch of kids how Sandy Dunes would sit up like a meerkat if you offered her a bit of hamburger, when I happened to look up.

There was a burgundy Chevy Suburban slowly pulling an aluminum horse trailer decorated with bunting and an enormous white banner with blue letters that said, "MAKE-A-WISH FOUNDATION OF OREGON" with the telltale wishbone tied with a ribbon logo. People started rushing to their cars to make room for the vehicle along our long, narrow driveway. At first, I didn't understand why the Make-A-Wish foundation would decorate a horse trailer like that, and I thought, *Wow, some kid is getting their wish today.* Then it hit me like a Mack truck. *You idiot! It's you! You're the kid! They tricked you!* I felt big tears welling up in my eyes and heat in my throat. *Don't cry. Whatever you do, don't cry in front of all these people.*

The truck and trailer slowly crept up our gravel driveway. I started walking towards it, knowing Dollie was inside but not able to believe that she actually was. I met it halfway down the driveway, and I went straight to the flip-down windows. I saw a dark head and eye peering at me. I burst into tears, sobbing unceremoniously and unabashedly. I released the handle on the window, and Dollie's shiny black head thrust out, nostrils flared, ears pricked forward, observing the excitement.

Mom came up behind me. "Whaddaya think, Boo? Huh?" I couldn't stop with the awkwardly loud sobs to say anything. Part of me was embarrassed, but most of me only had eyes for Dollie. This was a dream come true.

The Suburban stopped in front of the house, and I opened the back door of the trailer. I walked in, and Dollie's head turned to look at me. She was a gorgeous, shiny black; her coat was dusted with gold sparkles and she was wearing a large collar of multicolored carnations. Her scarlet halter and lead had brass buckles, and on each side of the halter there were brass plates engraved with "Make-A-Wish Foundation of Oregon" and "Intimidating Dollie/July 3, 1994." I untied her lead and we walked out of the trailer. She almost leapt down onto the gravel, head and tail held high. Everyone approached to pet her and bring her carrots and apple slices from the buffet table. The Make-A-Wish volunteers were there, and they gave a speech about the process involved in getting Dollie for me, and all the people who were a part of it. They also presented me with a new saddle, blanket, brushes, and some odds and ends for Dollie–it was so much more than I ever imagined. I forgot all about the last 15 months.

We arranged for Dollie to be kept at a neighbor's barn for a while. There was an arena there, and I'd go up every day to ride that summer. The show saddle that Make-A-Wish provided was gorgeous. It was a medium dark brown, decorated with silver plates on all the flaps, cantle, buckles, and a little disc on top of the horn. It was the most beautiful thing I'd ever seen. Sharon donated an old show bridle and breastcollar that matched. After I'd had at them with some silver polish, Dollie was the most beautiful show horse I'd ever seen. She was an absolute joy. She had an easy, side-to-side sort of jog and a slow, swinging lope. She could change leads with a small "cluck" and a nudge, and her showmanship almost required no lead. She had been trained with manners—she never fought me for the grass on the ground, and would respond to the slightest lift on the bit by rounding her back and powering through her gaits.

After a few months, we moved her back to our farm, where we'd set up an old stall in the barn. A friend of Sharon's gave me some thick rubber mats, and I arranged them all like a puzzle over the concrete floor of the stall. I cleaned out the rest of the barn, clearing the aisles out from decades of accumulating junk, dust, and straw. I arranged nails in the wall to hang all the halters, headstalls, and leads. I put up a whiteboard to keep track of her vet, farrier, and 4-H dates. I kept the workout saddles on a couple of sawhorses because I didn't have any saddleracks, and the showsaddle in a quilted saddlebag in the house.

Dollie had shown up just in time for the 4-H fair season. At the end of July, she and I packed up and arrived at the Washington County Fairgrounds with the rest of my 4-H club to show. We won Showmanship, Western Horsemanship, and English Equitation. We made the Finals class in both Western Horsemanship and English Equitation, and qualified for State that year. I was both wildly excited and terrified at how comfortable I was with her, and how my performances were suddenly competitive. I wasn't intimidated anymore by the other kids around me. I had just as much edge as they did.

In August, I discovered I had a problem. Mom had finally convinced me to go to Camp UKANDU with Travis. Now that I was in remission, I wasn't as afraid to go somewhere without Dr. Wolff being nearby. Camp UKANDU was a week long summer camp hosted by the local chapter of the American Cancer Society. It was designed specifically for kids with cancer and their siblings. They have full time nurses and oncologists on site to take care of any issues that might come up, but otherwise, it's just a week of outrageous fun where it doesn't matter a lick to anyone if you're bald. The problem was, camp and the state 4-H shows overlapped. Luckily, the camp directors allowed me to leave camp for three days, compete, and then return. Problem solved.

The first week of August arrived, and I started riding like crazy. I practiced and practiced. Dollie and I worked on longe line, showmanship, and equitation. We did patterns, drills, and more. I was able to get a few lessons from a trainer. I diligently polished all the leather and silver. I organized my show clothes. I was definitely going with the red silk double-breasted jacket with the sequins. It looked very dramatic. If there was a day I didn't ride, I would take Dollie to the arena and let her loose to play on her own. She'd buck and snort and roll maniacally. Then, when I held up her red halter and clucked to her, she'd trot right up to me, perfectly behaved.

Camp started on the third Sunday in August. State started the following Wednesday. Mom drove Travis and I out to Yamhill where the camp would be held. It was the same camp where I'd gone to outdoor school the year before my diagnosis–that all seemed so long ago, as if it was another life. We were assigned to our cabins. I was in with the "younger teen" girls, also known as the "2As." I felt instantly secure because Kaylee and Patsy were both there.

"Hi, Kaylee! Hi, Patsy!" I yelled as I passed the nurse's cabin.

"You can't call them that," said a girl behind me. "You have to call them by their camp names." I looked at her.

"Camp names? Why? What are their camp names?" Why would you have different names at camp anyway? I didn't understand the point.

"That's Meow," she pointed to Kaylee, then to Patsy, "and that's Mosquito." Meow and Mosquito said that Dr. Wolff came out for a day or two and that there would always be one of the doctors around. I saw Dr. Norman and felt that if anything could go wrong, I wouldn't want anyone else to take care of me other than these people. One of my cabin counselors I knew from the X-ray department. She had been taking pictures of my chest for the last year. Her camp name was Cosmo. Later, we met the 2Bs. One of the counselors was named Thumper. All us girls in 2A thought he was just so totally hot, and the other girls would try to tease him and flirt with him. I kept back, though, remembering all-too-clearly the incident with the college boys at Holly's house.

There was so much to do at camp, it was amazing. We did archery. We went fishing. We did arts and crafts. We sang songs. After my first day, I wished I'd listened to Mom and Dr. Wolff in the first place and gone the first time I was diagnosed. I'd missed out on two summers at camp already. On the first night, at camp-fire, a guy appeared in the firelight from out of the darkness in full Native American headdress. As he walked around the fire and found a place to stand, leaning on his staff, the fire burst with a loud "poof" and flash of white light. I'd never seen anything like it. I was in awe. Of course, he was white, so the illusion wasn't complete, but he did a pretty good job of convincing me. His name was, appropriately, Chief.

"The Great Spirit beckons us all into this sacred place..." he began.

A girl leaned over and whispered in my ear. "Every year it's the same." Her name was Bailey.

"How many years have you been here?" I whispered. Chief kept talking.

"I've been here since I was eight."

"Wow, how have you been able to come for so long?" Camp UKANDU stipulated that as long as you are on treatment, you and your siblings could come to camp. After remission, you could go for two years, or, if you had a permanent disability from your treatment, you could go until you were eighteen.

"I'm blind in one eye."

I didn't know what to say to that. I didn't have any permanent effects, except for that ringing in my ears which didn't quite seem comparable to blindness. "Oh," I whispered. I realized for a moment that it never mattered how bad my situation was, there was always going to be someone else who had it worse. Bailey definitely had it worse. Then I turned my attention back to Chief. He told a story about how the Native Americans would wrap their most precious items in the color red. He had a long staff with a dream catcher on the top, and around the staff were wound threads of varying colors, but the first and the last were red.

"That is why, tonight, we will wrap you all in red, for each of you is most precious to us and to everyone else who knows you." One of the counselors pushed a wheelbarrow into the circle. In it was a sapling. "We come from many different places, moons from here, and we are all different people. But when we come together we can do wonderful things." Everyone was supposed to bring a cup of dirt from their backyards so we could plant a new tree at the camp that had a part of all of us in it. We were called by cabin to go forward, and the staff members would wrap us in a red sweatshirt with the Camp UKANDU chief logo on the front. Kaylee wrapped me in mine. Then, we walked into the darkness toward our cabin. The whole thing had been very magical. I wished Chris could've seen it, but he was still in Maryland.

On Wednesday morning, Mom's white Toyota Camry pulled into camp. I threw my stuff in the backseat and climbed in.

"Sharon came and picked up Dollie today," she said. "She got your tack, your clothes, and everything." We headed for Salem.

I'd never been to the Oregon State Fairgrounds before. It felt enormous to me, like I was a wee guppy and it was the ocean. Eventually we were able to find the Washington County team aisle. I went down the rows of stalls until I found Dollie's. She was in there, haunches toward the door, dozing. There was a large blue ribbon on the front of the stall that said "Washington County State Qualifier" on it. I thought, *Well, we've already got one blue ribbon, and I'm happy with just that.*

The woman who was in charge of the team instructed us to go register and get my number. Mom and I set off for the main arena. As we left the mild shade of the horse barn and stepped into the hot summer light, I saw kids were out longeing and exercising their horses everywhere. Horses and riders were exiting the main arena when we found it. There were some classes going on already.

There was a booth labeled "Show Office." I walked up to the counter and said, "Lindsey VanDyke."

"Horse's name?" a man asked.

"Intimidating Dollie."

"Oh, you're already checked in." I stopped for a second, surprised. Had Sharon checked me in somehow? I didn't think so.

"Who checked me in?" I asked.

The guy looked at me like I was an idiot. "*You* did."

"No, I didn't. I just got here, like, ten minutes ago."

"Well, I show you're already checked in."

Mom piped up, "Wait a minute. We really did just get here. There must be some error."

The guy looked really tired. "OK. You're Lindsey VanSlyke, from Klamath County…"

Mom and I interrupted together, "No, Lindsey Michelle Van*Dyke*. From Washington County."

Understanding dawned on his face. "Oh, OK. Hang on a second. It looks like your number was given to her. We'll page her."

We waited by the show office until a woman and daughter showed up carrying a number. We got it all straightened out. Lindsey VanSlyke gave me my number, and the guy gave the other Lindsey her real number.

Mom said, "That is so weird that your name is Lindsey VanSlyke! How do you spell Lindsey?"

The girl, who was about my age said, "L-I-N-D-S-E-Y."

I said, "Oh my God, that's how I spell it! No one spells it with an E!"

She looked at me knowingly. "I know! They always spell it with an A."

"I know! Spell it how it sounds, why don'tcha?" I said.

"Tell me about it," she said as she rolled her eyes.

"God, that's so weird that we have almost the same name. What's your middle name?" I asked.

"Michelle."

Mom and I looked shocked. "No way!" Mom shouted. She looked at Mrs. VanSlyke. "What's your name?" she asked.

"Linda. It's nice to meet you."

Mom's and my mouths were agape. "Oh my God!" Mom exclaimed. "That's *my* name!" We sat around for a few minutes more, discussing the wild impossibilities of this many coincidences. In the end, we agreed that Lindsey and I needed to pose with our horses together after Showmanship the next day. We just happened to be in the same class.

Sharon met up with us that afternoon to practice Showmanship with me. Then I needed to exercise Dollie, so she critiqued my equitation.

Early the next morning, we were at the fairgrounds again. I was grooming Dollie and spraying her with fly repellant and ShowSheen. She was glistening by the end of it. Sharon arrived with a halter bag in hand.

"Here, punkin. I want you to use this today." I unzipped the halter bag, and inside was Sharon's silver show halter. It was a lot prettier than my nylon halter.

"Wow," I breathed. "Thank you." I went to dress for my class and put on makeup. I had a half hour to warm up.

As I stood at the in-gate, I went through a checklist. Number? Check. Horse? Check. Clothes? Check. I scanned Dollie for any dust or shavings that might be sticking to her coat or hooves. She looked good. Sharon had oiled Dollie's face and taken out the braid in her tail. As I coiled the flat leather lead in my left, gloved hand, I looked out over the other competitors. This was a big class. All the horses looked good. All the competitors looked good. I started to panic. I couldn't beat these kids. I suddenly felt a lot of pressure. This horse had been a gift to me, and I needed to prove to everyone that I deserved that gift, and that I deserved all the money that was being spent for us to be here. Pressure.

The gate opened, and before it revealed my face, I plastered the huge, fake Showmanship smile on my face and glided through the dirt, Dollie at my right shoulder. I showed like I'd never showed before. I never lost eye contact with the judges. I walked straighter than I'd ever walked. We executed our pattern. Right in the middle, Dollie flinched on a haunch turn. We recovered, but I knew it was over. We took our place in line while we waited for the other kids to finish their patterns. I set Dollie up perfectly square on all four feet and continued to watch the judges. While they were watching the other kids do their patterns, I'd relax my face for a while. We waited and waited. Finally, the judges started their final walk-throughs. As one came up to Dollie and me, I smiled so big that my teeth were taking over my face. I stayed out of his way while he examined her. Maybe I could squeak in with a blue after all.

"Will you please set up your horse?" the judge asked me. What? I looked down at her feet. She was resting her back left hoof. I groaned inwardly. *Oh, Dollie! You can't fall asleep like that.* Setting her up again was useless. She was zoned out, and the situation just got worse. In the end, I was able to get her pretty square again, and the judge moved on. After they were done with everyone, the announcer instructed us to relax and wait for the results. Most of the kids stopped smiling and let their horses sniff the dirt and such. I didn't. Sharon always told us to never stop showing. Ever. I stood there, stiff as a board, with the smile glued to my face. I watched Dollie's feet. She kept resting that left foot. I was starting to get mad at her. She knew better than this!

When they started announcing the awards (they always started with the lowest scores), I finally relaxed a little. I knew we'd delivered a lame performance. I just hoped our names weren't announced first. They weren't. After they'd awarded quite a few reds, I thought we might be able to eke by into the blues. Just as I was thinking that, they announced me. "NUMBER 143, LINDSEY VANDYKE AND INTIMIDATING DOLLIE...RED." Damn. I was angry, then. I'd been given this beautiful horse, and I still wasn't pulling off good results when it mattered. I took my red ribbon from the steward and left the building. I didn't wait around for Mom and everyone. I just went back to the Washington County stalls and released Dollie into her box and gave her some hay.

As I was affixing the loser red ribbon to the stall door, everyone showed up, trying to console me, saying, "These things happen...not every class is winnable," and "You did great; after all, you haven't even had Dollie for two months yet," or "Next year you'll get it." But the bottom line was that Showmanship is a class where they were watching *me*. Dollie was a tool, but the class was about *me*. How well *I* could show. How well *I* could master the horse. And I blew it. I should've watched her feet. I should've handled her flinch better. I should've done everything better. And I wanted to show with the pros? Yeah right. If I couldn't cut it in *4-H*, there was no way I'll make it against all the kids with twenty-thousand-dollar horses, one-thousand-dollar-a-month training programs, and pedigrees up the wazoo.

I never took that picture with Lindsey VanSlyke, and later felt very guilty. I can be so selfish sometimes.

On the drive back to camp, Mom tried to take the "tough love" approach to my losing attitude. While she was lecturing me on "being positive" and how my "attitude is unbecoming" and blah blah blah, I zoned out. The lecture just made me feel worse, like more of a loser, even more "not good enough" if that were possible. I never understood the idea that if you felt bad about yourself or were angry about something, adults always wanted you to "get your act together" and "quit having an attitude." I didn't understand why it wasn't OK just to run the gamut of emotion. Getting yelled at for feeling something seemed to me a waste of energy.

Finishing off the week at camp cured my attitude. The last night, at campfire, we had another visit from Chief. That day, we had made "wishboats" and "wishbundles." The boats were big pieces of bark decorated with flowers, stones, leaves and any other pretty memento we'd found or made. We would then light little votives, set them on the boats, and send them off downriver that night. Our wishbundles were prayers, or thoughts or fears that we had. We wrote them down and bundled sticks around the rolled up piece of paper with a red ribbon. Then we gave them to our counselors. That night, we sat around the campfire, holding our wishboats and looking at our wishbundles in a big basket at Chief's feet.

"We have gathered together again tonight to make an offering to the Great Spirit," Chief began. He picked up the basket. "We now release ourselves from the burdens of life, and ask the Great Spirit to be with us and keep our prayers." He dumped the all the bundles into the fire, which blazed with sparks and white light, punctuated by an occasional "poof!" I watched my thoughts and prayers go up in red sparks and faint smoke, disappearing into the black of the night forest. I felt relief that they were all going to God.

Cosmo gathered us all around and gave us candles for our wishboats. We lit them and walked down to the riverbank and set them in the water. With a slight push, they set off, dodging rocks and swirling eddies. Some of them capsized. Some of the candles were doused. I watched mine float away until I couldn't distinguish it from any of the other boats out there. Then I dashed from the riverbank up to the bridge, overlooking the whole river. It was the most beautiful thing I'd ever seen. The river was a winding path of light in an ocean of blackness.

"Every year we do the same thing," Bailey said walking up next to me, "and every year it is still the most beautiful thing in the world." I felt utterly and infinitely peaceful at that moment. Nothing could touch me. I was surrounded by life. I looked over at a cluster of girls, clinging to Thumper, sobbing.

Little did I know that half a dozen staff members were scrambling up and down the riverbanks putting out the candles around the bend where none of us could see, so we didn't start any forest fires.

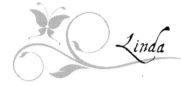

Linda

She was going into high school, and I thought, Good, she's finally going to finish off being a kid. *I was worried a little about her hair still being so short and how she might deal with it. I told the administration that Dr. Wolff had ordered her to avoid contact sports and that they would really have to watch her at first, especially in PE, because of her lung.*

I thought her yearbook picture was really cute, with her hair so short.

When I'd been admitted to Jesuit High School—no small feat—the first person I called was Dr. Wolff, interrupting his dinner. But I was too excited, and I knew that he would be impressed. And he was. I was proud of myself, but mostly satisfied that he was proud of me.

After I returned from camp, we went to Freshman Orientation and Registration. I got my locker—it's funny how you can remember some things so lucidly. I still remember that it was locker #225 in Perry Hall and its combination was 38-28-18. We met with the Principal to discuss my hair situation. It had barely started to grow again, and I only had a couple millimeters' worth. Mom was concerned that the other kids would make fun of me and asked if it was all right to break school policy about hats for a little while. We had abandoned the wig, because after 9 months it looked pretty ratty, and Mom didn't want to buy another one. I didn't want to *wear* one, for that matter. Mr. Patterson suggested that since Jesuit's dress code stipulates "no hats in classrooms" I'd likely draw more attention to myself if I did wear a hat, and that if I could grin and bear it it'd blow over. Then he said, "If you have any problems, you just let me know. But we won't do anything to draw attention to it. I'll make sure each of your teachers gets a note. Which teachers do you have?" I handed over my class schedule.

"OK, Nagel, Renshaw, Hazel…" He looked up at me. "Ooh, Hazel. Boy, you don't screw around in *that* guy's class." I was suddenly scared. Who were these people? What would they make me do? Would I be able to keep up? I'd missed almost three hundred days of school in the last three years. My placement exam scores weren't that great. I had to take Algebra again. Holly had been put into some accelerated classes, but I wasn't. Would I fit in? I was coming from a school that had a total student body of about one hundred, and starting at a school with a student body of one thousand. Plus, this Hazel guy already sounded like some kind of a draconian megalomaniac, and I hadn't even met him yet.

I went back to see Wolff in the clinic before school started. I had to have a physical for Jesuit, and it was time for a chest X-ray. Cosmo from camp took my X-ray that day, and when I brought it back to Dr. Wolff, he put it up on the light board with me. I didn't know how he could be so sure he wasn't looking at tumors. I made out my ribs, heart, stomach, and intestines, but everything else looked so *cloudy*.

"Dense things, like bone, show up as white. Less dense things and airspace show up dark," Dr. Wolff explained. I could see the outline of what little breasts I had in the X-ray: faint, white, half-moon looking things over my ribs. Down lower in my abdomen, Dr. Wolff pointed to a dark spot amidst all the white. "Do you know what that is?" He asked, grinning. I looked. Black. That meant less dense or airspace. Was it gas? It must be, but I wasn't sure. And I kind of didn't want to talk about my gas with him.

"No," I said, looking at him, expecting an answer.

"Wait a few hours. You'll know," he said, grinning, as he took the films off the light board. On my physical for Jesuit, he wrote under the hair category "alopecia." I asked him what that meant. "It means your hair has fallen out," he answered matter-of-factly. *What a fabulous word.* I expected him to write a ton of stuff on it, but the only other thing he added was "no collision sports." I looked at it.

"No collision sports. Why?" I asked him.

"You need to protect your kidney. It's the only one you've got now, so I don't want you catching an elbow in the kidney while you're playing basketball, or getting nailed while you're in a rugby scrum." It made sense. I was highly motivated to stay off the kidney transplant list.

On the first day of school, I had mixed emotions. I was glad that Holly had been accepted, too, so I'd have one friend at least. We were the only two kids from our school going to Jesuit. Everyone else in our 8th grade class was going to Forest Grove or Banks High Schools. That made me want to go there, too, so I could have some friends, but Mom and Dad were pretty adamant. They wanted a guarantee that I'd be going to college. It was quite a trek to Jesuit—eighteen miles each way from the farm, about a forty-five minute drive or a ninety minute bus ride.

The first day started off on the wrong foot with PE where I found myself having to change clothes with 25 strangers who were healthy and unmarked. I didn't want them to see my scars. As luck would have it, my assigned locker was right in the middle of the room. So I loitered, trying to wait until most of the girls had left before quickly changing and rushing out to catch up. I shuddered at the idea of fitness testing. I would surely fail. My PE teacher was a balding, stocky, British man whose legs betrayed him as a serious soccer player. Second period was algebra. My teacher was a Welsh soccer coach. Third period was Fine arts. I was supposed to have drama, but the classroom was in a secret place and I couldn't find it. I ended up embarrassing myself in front of a bunch of seniors by accidentally going to the advanced drama class. When I realized my mistake, I froze. I was scared of the seniors–they were all so *big*. Then there was lunch, which was a whole other drama in and of itself. Jesuit had two lunches. If you had fourth period in certain halls, you went to first lunch. If fourth period was in one of the other halls, you went to second lunch. It was very confusing. I had first lunch but no one to sit with. I tried my best to be bold and sit with people at tables with empty chairs, but I'd get a lot of weird looks. Then I'd remember, *Oh, right. I'm bald.* It took months to make friends.

Fourth period was the dreaded English with Hazel. I sweated through that class. Almost everything you did could land you a detention, which at Jesuit was known as JUG—kids said it was an acronym for "Justice Under God." In his class, if he called on you when you raised your hand, and you didn't introduce yourself, JUG. If you used the word *like* as a conjunction and didn't catch and correct yourself, JUG. If you weren't in your seat, books open and in the process of taking notes when the second bell rang, JUG.

And on, and on, and on the list of punishable activities grew as the year wore on. Though there was no slack anywhere, I have to admit the class had one redeeming factor. He had the sharpest, most caustic wit I'd ever heard, and I laughed a lot in spite of my sheer terror. I fully expected he'd make me cry at some point— probably in front of everyone else—and that fear turned out to not be unfounded. *So,* I thought to myself as I walked out of his classroom one day, *I'll be failing PE* and *English this year.*

Fifth period was world history, which I hated and which was nondescript. Sixth period was Spanish–which I knew I'd love. Seventh period was keyboarding, which I loathed for all but one reason: I had been assigned to a seat next to a boy, on whom I had an immediate and instant super-crush.

Between bells, we had five minutes to transfer between classes, which I found outrageously nerve-wracking since the campus was exponentially bigger than Visitation's, and the idea of running like scared cattle was scary in and of itself. My biggest fear was needing to stop off at my locker to swap out books, being unable to get it to unlock, and getting caught there trying to open it when that second bell rang. JUG.

Try as I might, I was unable to make friends for lunch, so I quit eating after a while. Instead, I'd go to the library and get ready for Hazel's class. After a few weeks, I wasn't even hungry anymore at lunchtime, and I'd make it through my day with no problems. Between my reduced-calorie diet and a stringent PE class that was killing me, I quickly shed all the water weight and extra fat I'd picked up while on treatment.

PE was dehumanizing. For the initial set of fitness tests, I didn't score better than a C on anything. Two dozen kids, who had all their own God-given giblets, who were school athletes, or who were just plain normal, surrounded me. My initial distance in the twelve-minute run was two and a half laps. Everyone beat me by a mile—even the asthmatics. Then, of course, when it came time for the sports (rugby, lacrosse, soccer, baseball, etc.), the teacher stuck me on the Stairmaster in the weight room. The only things I participated in that year were fitness testing and the sections on track, weight training, and folk dancing (yes, *folk dancing*). The rest of my PE year was spent on the Stairmaster. I had buns of steel.

PE was a blessing, though, too. I met my first two friends there, and they were the closest people to me through high school. One day, I was wearing my T-shirt with all the different horses on it, and another girl with shocking red hair said, "I really like your shirt." She sparked a mini-conversation between the two of us for a few minutes, that would lead to a long lasting friendship. She deserves a lot of credit. It probably took a lot of guts to talk to the bald girl. Her name was Marie. On another day, I was climbing the Stairmaster, when the teacher brought in another girl and put her on the stationary bike next to me. She introduced herself as Kendall and we talked the whole period about how we were stuck in there, and why. She was an artist, so I was excited we had something important in common right away. Although I would come to find out that she was much better at drawing than I. She wasn't in there as much as me, because she was allowed to play contact sports.

All in all, though, freshman year sucked. People would make remarks like, "So, what kind of statement are you trying to make with that hair? Or should I say, *lack* of hair?" or "So, are you a lesbian or something? I mean, why would you butch your hair like that if you weren't?" or just plain "Why do you shave your head?" Initially, I just ignored the comments and questions and kept on about my own business. But it continued. Finally, I decided that ignoring it wouldn't make it go away. So I opted for the truth, figuring it'd get around eventually. Maybe then it all would stop. One day, I was sitting at my desk in Mr. Hazel's class, minding my own business, and the kid in front of me whipped around in his chair.

"So...like, why do you cut your hair like that? You a lesbian or somethin'?"

I only had a very vague idea of what a lesbian really was, but I was pretty sure I wasn't one. I rolled my eyes and mustered the courage to talk back. I stared him in the eyes and said, "I don't *cut* my hair like this. It *fell* out because I had *cancer*." He paled and turned around front again really fast. It gave me a lot of satisfaction to scare him like that. So the truth worked.

But if I wasn't dodging glances from people, I felt like I was floundering no matter what I did. Hazel's class made me neurotic. Considering I'd only been punished at school a couple of times in my entire life, I lived in constant fear of the JUG thing whenever I was within fifty feet of that classroom. However, the worst part of freshman year had nothing to do with school at all.

In late September, I was up to see Dr. Wolff for a regularly scheduled CT. Those things always take forever and, of course, aren't always pleasant. Anytime they injected the contrast dye for the abdominal scans, I seemed to react worse and worse. This time, it caused me to feel so hot and violently nauseous I started to scream in pain. They stopped the scan and someone rushed in. "Tell me what you feel," he said.

"I'm too hot! Too hot! I need Benadryl!" I retched and added, "I'm going to throw up on you!"

He brought me one of the little banana shaped emesis basins, which I always find insulting. I can fill one of those up in half a heave. "It's not supposed to make you feel like that," he posited. "It should just make you feel a little warm…"

I was sobbing by this time, my stomach in agony. "Yes, I *know*," I said, trying desperately to control myself and not grab him by the throat, "but I'm telling *you* that it *is* making me feel bad. I…need… Benadryl. Twenty-five milligrams should be enough. Or else you'll be carrying me out." They didn't have any on hand, so they had to order it, and I sat there for God knows how long before it came to me. He pushed it through my port—which I'd decided to keep until I passed the cure date—and I immediately cooled down and the nausea disappeared into sleep.

The Benadryl wore off as the rest of my appointments progressed. By this time I was pretty good at fighting the sleep effects if I had to. Everything continued to look good, too. No tumors. The scar tissue that had scared us all so badly seemed unchanged. When everything was done, we went up to 14A for a quick hello.

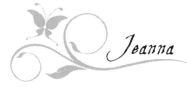

Jeanna

I brought her back up to visit 14A and she found out Chris was there. Dr. Wolff told Linda that this was not a good time to be developing her friendship with Chris. I felt bad reintroducing them. I remember his mom sitting in the corner of his room, knitting or crocheting or something. She had this peaceful smile on her face, and I thought, Oh, this is pretty routine for them. *But that smile never changed the whole time we were there. That was what she put on to make it work for him. It was like a Mr. Potato Head smile. One that can be turned around from a frown to a smile and just stay that way.*

When we walked onto the ward, I went to the nurse's desk to ask for Karen and/or Denise. While I was waiting, I recognized movement out of the corner of my right eye. I looked over, and saw Chris's mom in the isolation room. I recognized the shadow of a tall boy behind the curtain. I left the nurses' desk to say hello.

"Hey, you guys!" I said, smiling big, as I walked into the room. Chris was unpacking. Sue was at the foot of the bed. "What're you in for?"

Chris looked down as he continued to unpack, while Sue looked right at me. Silence hung in the air for awhile. "We've had a relapse," she said quietly, almost sweetly. I looked up at her, eyes wide. Here was a woman of infinite patience. I gasped. *No.* I looked at them both, wildly, not knowing what to say. Should I play it positive or be serious? I opted for the positive route.

"Don't worry. Everything will work out fine." Yeah, that sounded good. That's what Rachel said to me the first night I'd been diagnosed, and she'd been right. I'm sure I sounded entirely patronizing. I smiled at them both. "How long will you be here?" I asked him. He said off and on for the next couple months. They were going to prepare him for a bone marrow transplant. "I'll come up and visit you after school some days, OK? I'll bring my friend Holly. We'll have some good times."

I told Mom what I'd found out. The next day, while waiting for the bus with Holly, I told her. She agreed to come up to OHSU with me to see him, since she knew him a little from the times she would visit me. We decided that every Monday after school would be a good start. One of our moms would pick us up from school on Mondays and take us up to OHSU for an hour or so. If Mom came with us, we could stay longer because she and Sue were pals and they'd go off together for coffee. Holly and I would bring stuff to do. Once, we brought The Farming Game. We'd had it for as long as I could remember, and I never did know how to play it. But it came with re-stickable stickers that had pictures of wheat, cows, combines, and corn on them. We'd stick them all over his Standley, and Holly would make like she was pulling on invisible overall straps and do farmer impressions. It'd make Chris laugh for a while if nothing else. He was always very polite and quiet. Some days, he was on drugs that made him almost totally incoherent; he would try valiantly to stay awake and play, but he would succumb in the end, and we'd tiptoe out.

He had beautiful, curly, dark blonde/light brown hair. He really was a handsome young man. I found myself devoted to our scheduled meetings once a week. Sometimes I would go by myself. Once, he was in the room where I had first been put in November 1991. He was in the exact same bed. I walked in, and he opened his eyes and smiled at me.

"H'llo," he said.

I smiled back. "Hey." I looked at his IV bag. It was wrapped up in a black garbage bag. "Why's it like that?" I asked, gesturing to the bag.

He sighed a little, and shrugged. "It's light sensitive. It won't work if it's in the light, so they cover it." I noticed the lights were off in his room, too. Mostly, when I would come alone, it wasn't a loud laugh fest. We would just talk to each other. I was comfortable with him. We understood each other, if only on the basal level that we had shared the same horrifying experiences. I would tell stories about funny things Holly and I would do while I was in the hospital, though. Sleepovers and throwing fruit snacks at the ceiling until they stuck. He laughed in disbelief at our antics. Once, we pondered the reality of children dying on the ward.

"I've heard commotion in the hallways a couple times during my stays," I said. "You know something bad is happening when someone comes and closes your door." He nodded. I had to keep talking, of course. I leaned in a little, sideways, and asked in a hushed tone, "How do you think they get them off the ward? You know…after?" I looked at him. It was an innocent question, I thought. He just looked back at me. After a long time, he said, "I don't know." And yet, my huge mouth wouldn't shut.

"Do you think they cover them up or just leave them uncovered? You know, like they're sleeping. I think seeing a covered bed is scarier than seeing someone rolling down the hall like they're sleeping. You know?"

"Yeah, maybe."

By then, I realized what I'd been talking about, and I changed the topics suddenly. "So, you wanna play The Farming Game?"

Around the time Chris relapsed, my cancer community was hit with another tragedy. Dr. Norman, the man of the Tasteful Ties, had died suddenly. I came home from school one day, and Mom told me. I was devastated. No more puns. No more tasteful ties. No more surrogate Dr. Wolff. *Oh, God, Dr. Wolff,* I thought. *What'll I do if he dies?* I was suddenly more afraid of the prospect of something happening to Dr. Wolff than I was aggrieved over Dr. Norman. That is, until *The Oregonian* printed an article about him. I sobbed while I read the quotes from patients and parents whose lives he'd touched and saved. I read about children he wasn't able to save, and about families that were just as thankful that he tried. About graduations he attended, rejoicing that the child in question was finished with treatment and moving on with life. I learned that he'd been instrumental in establishing Camp UKANDU. The photograph they used of him was perfect. Dr. Norman peering over his shoulder with an open mouthed grin. That's how I'll always remember him.

But the article made me think. What if Dr. Wolff hadn't been able to save me? What if something went wrong and I'd just up and died? What would Mom and Dad have done? I asked Dad as much one evening and was shocked by his simple response. "We probably would have sued him. Or the hospital. Or both." Aghast, I demanded to know why. It seemed to me that cancer was a pretty sneaky Pete, and even the best treatments don't always work. His answer was simple but unacceptable to me. "Because you were our little girl. And they told us that cure rates were good."

What high schooler's life isn't fraught with complications? Mine was no different. Although, I suspected that the types of complications I dealt with were unique to my age group. Shortly after Dr. Norman's death, I was riding home from OHSU with Mom. We had just been up for a clinic appointment and a visit to Chris and Sue, when Mom said something I'll never forget.

"Linds, I want to talk to you about something."

Oh, God. This wasn't going to be some kind of sex talk, was it? Ick.

"What?" I asked, not turning my head to look at her. Beaverton Hillsdale Highway rolled by.

"I think we should have a talk about Chris."

Wait, a sex-talk about Chris? Now it was getting weird. I looked at her, frowning.

"What about Chris?" I asked, narrowing my eyes, with catlike reflexes ready for any defense.

"Well...I'm not sure...really...if it's a good idea for you to be spending so much time with him..."

I was shocked. "What! Why?" Now I was watching her intently. She looked calmly forward, piloting the car down the highway.

"Well, because his disease is very different from yours. It's much more difficult to cure."

"*So?*" I was not getting the point. But in my defense, she was not being direct. "It's just that...well, I don't want you to get hurt. You know," she finished. I scoffed indignantly at her, not sure of what I should say, or of what I could say for that matter. She wanted me to stay away from him because he had a more complicated disease than I did? It didn't make any sense. I knew what it was like to while away the hours on 14A. It made sense that I should be near him.

"Get hurt? From what? And then what? Just leave him up there by himself? Why? There's no one up there his age. I was the closest there was, and you saw the patient board. All the kids in there right now are, well, *kids.*" I looked out the window again. I was furious. If I looked right at her I might start to cry, and I couldn't stand to do that in front of her. But it was preposterous! She expected me to leave one of my kindred spirits behind during a time when otherwise he might be spending hours alone? Besides, he was hours from his home. Often, no one was there with him. His parents had their hands full: one kid in the hospital and still two at home to take care of. We'd never faced a challenge like that. We lived so close. "I'm not doing it. I'm not going to stop seeing him. How would we have felt if our friends had done that to us? Just quit coming over because I had a disease and they didn't? One that was more complicated than anything they'd ever had? It's stupid." It took all night for me to calm down.

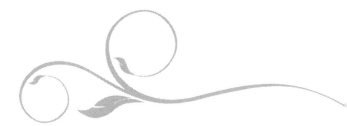

Life and school went ever onward. One day, I was at my locker getting books for Hazel's class, and two boys were sitting on the floor a few lockers down. One of them looked up and said, "Hey! Hey, you!" I turned to look down at him, perplexed. Nobody talked to me except the teachers and the two odd friends I'd managed to make so far. But especially boys didn't talk to me. This kid looked like trouble.

"Hey, would you go out with my friend here?" The other kid looked up at me. Both of them smiled comically, almost maniacally. I examined them for a few seconds, waiting for the punch line. Maybe this time it would be something along the lines of, "I think you're pretty—pretty funny looking that is!" You know, a real scream. Like I hadn't heard that one before. Anyway, regardless of punch lines, there was no way this could be a real proposition. I didn't have any hair for God's sake! How could anyone find me attractive? I shrugged at them, shut my locker, and stalked off to the library, laughing darkly to myself, *Oh, yeah. Right.* Later, I wondered if there had been a chance that he was being honest.

Christmas break arrived. I had never been more relieved to be out of school. I planned to spend the vacation primarily with the horse. I'd pulled off her shoes for the winter so her feet could spend some time in the mud, and if it snowed she would be in less danger of slipping and falling. There was no shortage of fun things to do. My 4-H club had a Christmas party. Holly's birthday was during the break. Christmas Eve we spent with Dad's side of the family. Christmas Day we spent with Mom's side of the family. For New Year's, Sharon was hosting a formal party. I was really excited for that one. One of my aunts had handed down a beautiful dark purple satin and lace dress that I really wanted to wear. My hair was coming in nicely, now, too. It was starting to curl. Plus, my lashes and brows were back in full. I was hoping to get some kind of a haircut so I didn't look like such a pin curled puffball. I'd heard the word "poodle" too often in the halls at school for it to be coincidence. If I could somehow shape my hair, maybe I'd consider myself more attractive, and that might lead to genuine interest from boys, not just mockery.

We had roughly two weeks off, and then two weeks after school resumed, final exams would take place. I'd never taken final exams before. I was paralyzed with fear of failure. I had never been a great tester to begin with, but Hazel might push me over the edge and I might just freeze right in the middle of the test. I decided to take advantage of my vacation to work on vocabulary for his class. He'd already informed us of the format and content of most of the exam.

On Christmas morning, we awoke to a beautiful day and had a spectacular morning filled with gifts and laughter and one of Mom's incredible breakfasts (I would not realize, until years later how "Norman Rockwell" our family was when it came to holidays). When I was putting "the haul" away in my room, the phone rang. Mom knocked on my door. "It's for you." She came in and handed me the cordless phone.

"Who is it?" I whispered. She just shrugged her shoulders on her way back out.

"Hello?" I asked.

"Hello!" It was a guy. He sounded vaguely familiar.

"Hi…" I said, still trying to figure out who it was.

"It's Chris!" Chris…Chris from keyboarding class? No…it didn't sound like him…wait… "Oh, my God, *Chris*! I totally didn't expect you to call! What's going on?" I flopped down on my bed. "I heard you were in transplant in LA. How's it going?" I was about to explode with excitement. I was so happy; I couldn't believe he was calling me. Of all people he might think of on Christmas morning, he was calling *me*. I loved him for it. He asked me how my Christmas was, and I described our morning and all the stuff I'd gotten. "What about you?" I asked.

"Oh, they don't allow stuff in here. You know how it is. Everything has to be sterile. But I got my laptop from Make-A-Wish, and I was able to bring it in with me in the beginning, so everything's great. It's amazing what this thing can do." He described teasing the nurses with e-mails and the procedures involved with a transplant: lots of radiation and heavy, large doses of chemo to get ready. His little brother was his marrow donor, and he'd just received the transplant a few days before.

"Wow, your brother gave you his marrow? A new life. That's the greatest Christmas gift, ever, huh?" I asked. I got silence on the other end for a response, so I plowed forward, as always, filling the quiet with noise, trying to move the conversation again. "So, do you have a window? How's sunny LA?" I asked.

"Oh, you can't see much from here…just more buildings. It sure is sunny a lot, though."

"How long until you can come back?" I asked.

"Three months total, and I've already been here for almost a month." I did the math in my head. February. I didn't say anything because I wanted to surprise him, but I was planning on meeting him when he returned, on the precise day and time he would start his new life.

"Three months!" I said. "Wow, that's a long time. I don't think I could handle staying in the hospital that long. I can't wait for you to come back." We chatted for a while longer until I could hear Mom yelling for me from the living room to get ready. My grandparents would be here soon. "Hey, Chris, I gotta go. My mom's calling for me. But I am so glad you called! It was so great talking to you!" I swear I was about ready to burst.

"Yeah, it was." He sounded a little despondent suddenly. I barely registered it.

"Hey, give me your number, and I'll call you back in a couple days, OK?" He gave me his digits and we hung up. Christmas 1994 was the best of my life.

In the end, there was a yeast.

On the night of January 2, I was in the basement studying vocab for Hazel's exam. The phone rang. For no good reason, a bolt of fear shot through my trunk as I felt a flashback to the night we heard about Dr. Norman. I could hear Mom answer the phone.

"Oh, hey, Kaylee! How are ya?" I froze, listening. Kaylee and Mom were friends. Whenever I was up there, they talked a lot. But she never called just to chat. Mom got suddenly quiet, and I could only hear mutterings of her side of the conversation. I suddenly felt scared, and I went into the office and shut the door. It was a much smaller room and somehow felt more secure. God, what if Dr. Wolff was dead this time? What if *he* had a heart attack? I didn't really think that was possible–the guy was a *stick*, for God's sake. But I couldn't shake the dread. I pretended to work on the computer, trying not to invent details, but I couldn't help it. Mom didn't come down. She didn't call me upstairs, either, so I started to relax. Kaylee must have just called about an appointment or something. *At eight o'clock at night? Are you stupid? It's something else, and you know it.*

Then, unexpectedly, someone knocked on the door. I hadn't heard anyone descend our creaky stairs. I looked up, filled with trepidation and that cold sharp feeling in my gut. Mom came in.

I stood up, clutching a packet of vocabulary papers.

"That was Kaylee on the phone."

I looked at her, terrified, trying to hide it under an impassive countenance. Her face changed subtly, but she kept it under control.

"Chris Mason died today."

I looked at her still, struggling for a response. Anything. But I was at a total loss. Anger. Shock. Despair. Nothing! Finally, it came. It was not what I expected. "*What?* Oh-ho yeah, right!" I said, looking down to shuffle my papers. "No. He's coming back in February."

"No, he's gone."

"No, he's not."

"Lindsey, Chris died. He got an infection, and they couldn't stop it."

I sighed and rolled my eyes as if this was the most inconvenient and disappointing thing in the world. Like he was purposely trying to trick me. I didn't know what else to do. I sat down in the chair at the computer.

I said nothing.

It took every ounce of control in my body to keep from going completely crazy at that moment. I wanted to shriek and throw things and tear the office apart. I wanted to destroy everything in front of me. I wanted to act out against the world, against God, against modern medicine. *To hell with school and final exams, and boys and all that. Forget CT scans and chest tubes; I can't stand facing this anymore.* I needed to break something, to scream, to do *something*. Anything to stop feeling like this. I felt as if my heart was being systematically stretched in every direction. My chest hurt. My head hurt. Everything hurt. My whole existence felt as though it was being slowly and deliberately torn in half—because it's more painful than a quick rip.

He was just a kid.

After I was able to get Mom to leave the room, I sobbed silently and thoroughly until I was parched. I couldn't stand the thought of anyone hearing me and coming in to try and comfort me. I didn't want anyone to see me cry. I just wanted to see Chris again. I just wanted to hear his voice.

He was just a kid.

So? We were both just kids and we got cancer. Shit happens.

Oh, yeah? Well what's so great about you? Why'd you live and he die? He was a nice boy. Everyone liked him. I pressed the heels of my hands on either side of my head and bit down on my tongue. Hard. Get. A. Grip.

I picked up the phone.

Holly answered.

"Chris is dead."

PART TWO: The AfterMath

I tortured myself for weeks, maybe months with unanswerable questions. When he called me, did he already know he was dying? Or did he call for plain old amusement? Did he like me? Is that why he called? Because I loved him. I mean, I didn't really know it because I was just a kid, but genuinely loved him. If he knew he was dying, how long had he known? Months? Days? Hours? Never? Had Dr. Stein told him as bluntly as she would have told me that he was going to croak? Did he go quickly, or did he suffer? Was his family around him or was he alone? Did he hate me for talking about death with him? Did he hate me for being ignorant? For being a self-centered little girl, who believed that because she had lived through her disease, that he would, too? Why didn't he get angry with me and tell me to shut up because death was his reality? I would've stepped into his place if I could have. I always felt he was a better person than me. If I had known he was dying, I would have wanted to be there. I would have wanted to stay with him, hold his pale hands, and be brushed by his soul as it left this world.

This must have been what Mom meant by "get hurt."

It was a yeast. A measly little bunch of yeasties. They got him. I understood some of the complexity of bone marrow transplants, and the immense risks they involved. But a yeast? I mean, they sell stuff *over the counter* to cure yeasts. I couldn't wrap my brain around the idea that something that small, insignificant, and curable could suddenly become something enormous, insurmountable, and untreatable. I accepted it in articles and stories I'd read, yet it was unacceptable when it involved *my friend.* I would pray at night, as I cried myself to sleep, for God to send me a dream about Chris. I just wanted to see him. To hear that he was well and happy. Even if my own subconscious conjured it up. So long as it was convincing. I would talk to the air about how I realized what an ass I was. How inconsiderate I could be. How self-centered. Often, if I was alone, I would find myself reduced to a heaving, sobbing, snotty shell of a person.

I dreaded the day of the funeral. Everyone said I had to go, that it would provide closure. I didn't really know what "closure" was supposed to mean. I wanted to wear black and cover my face with a black veil. I wanted the world to know I was in the worst pain of my life, but Mom wouldn't let me out of the house with any black on. Holly came with us. On the early morning drive down, I couldn't think about anything. Looking out the window, I watched the Oregon countryside roll by under a bright January sun as we passed through small towns on our way to his small town. I looked up at the front seat, thinking how weird it was that both of my parents were coming with me. God, why wasn't I old enough to drive? I didn't want them with me today. In so many ways, all of this felt entirely surreal. Perhaps everything that had happened this last week was a series of nightmares, and we were really going to go to his house and he'd be there ahead of schedule, with his new marrow. Cured. Then everyone would say, "Fooled you!" and it would be funny.

When we arrived at the church, I got out of the car and stood in the early chill looking up at the steeple. If this was a joke, it was getting elaborate.

"Are you ready for this?" I asked Holly.

"Are you?" she asked me.

"No."

We walked around to the entrance of the church, and all along the breezeway, at every pillar, were Boy Scouts. They stood as stock-still and determined as the men who guarded the Tomb of the Unknown Soldiers at Arlington National Cemetery. I walked between them, cringing under the straight, icy stares of these young boys, and some of them were indeed very young. They did not move. They did not speak. They barely breathed. Finally, I entered the church thankful for the reprieve from the baleful glares of the Boy Scouts, only to meet another awful sight. Chris's family. His dad, mom, sister, and brother. Of course, I greeted Sue and she introduced me to everyone else. The kids nodded politely, and his Dad shook my hand. Then I stood there, dumbly, looking at all of them. There was nothing I could say. What *do* you say to a family whose oldest son just died? I had learned over the last few days to loathe people who said, "I'm sorry." I could not grasp what on earth they were sorry about; this had nothing to do with them. I would not insult this family with such trite filler.

I looked from face to face. I saw the parts of his mother that were in Chris. I saw the traits that he got from his father. His brother was like a younger version of him. Exactly. As I looked at his sister, I noticed something gray behind them. Oh, God. It was the casket. They had put him *in a casket*. I was horrified. But I wished they would open it so I could see him. And he would be alive and well. I just knew it.

But the casket was closed and I couldn't stand to be near it. I excused myself and we migrated to one of the rear pews in the church. All the time I was turning things over in my head: I was the girl who lived. *Why?* During the whole funeral ceremony, I wondered about this. What was the reason I had lived while such a perfectly worthy child had died? What had I contributed to anything? All I had ever done my whole life was consume resources of one sort or another. I figured there sure as hell better be a purpose for me now. If I had to be stripped of the company of someone so fine as Chris, I had better be here to do something phenomenal for God or humanity or whatever. I'd better save someone else's life someday to make up for the one I'd lost this year.

I looked at the little program and read through a 1936 W.H. Auden poem called "Funeral Blues." It described how when someone dies, you're supposed to create silence–shut the clocks off, unplug the phones and quiet the dog. However, what I really wanted was noise. I wished a marching band would go by so no one could hear me sob. I didn't want people to hear me because I didn't want them to try and comfort me. They couldn't. I just wanted to grieve in peace. Auden also suggested that one is supposed to put bows on the "public doves." I had no idea if there were actually such things as public doves or if it was some kind of metaphor. If these doves were a metaphor, it was lost on me. If they weren't a metaphor, who's job would it be to catch them and put the bows on them? I don't know where Auden was from, but I was pretty sure my hometown didn't have any doves. We had a lot of Canadian geese, though, and it would be a far messier job to try and put bows on *them*. When I reached the end of Auden's last stanza, the very last line stopped my breath:

I thought that love would last forever: I was wrong.

Boy was I *ever* wrong. How could I be so stupid? How could I be so egocentric? It was easy, sometimes, for people to say to me, "Oh, you had cancer? Well, it wasn't that big a deal—you survived!" and sometimes I fell victim to that same line of thought. But the truth of it is that it *is* a big deal, and sometimes you *don't* survive. How could I not have seen this coming?

I looked around at everyone else in the church. These were his family, his friends. I had only known a miniscule sliver of who he was, and shared a tiny part of his life. As I listened to the eulogies, I learned more about him during his funeral than I had learned about him in all those hours together. Where he was born, when his birthday was, the names of his family members, activities he loved, people he loved, things he did. He earned his Eagle in an unheard of short period of time. I marveled at my stupidity. *My ignorance.* How could I not have asked these questions? It all seemed so simple all of a sudden. And I had failed to do any of it. I vowed to never take advantage of another human being for the rest of my life. I would not repeat this mistake.

Then it was over. Only the family would be allowed at the cemetery. We were asked to proceed to the reception. Then they sang the closing hymn "City of God." I hated that song from that day forward. "Awake from your slumber," my ass. "Arise from your sleep," huh? *Hey, God! Ya wanna rub it in a little more? Huh? Do ya? We aren't talking about* sleeping *here. This isn't a nap!*

As I was having my mental argument with God, they folded the stark white pall, and the bearers gathered around the gray casket. They wheeled it up the aisle and out of the church. I watched it approach me, and horror chilled me to the bone. I froze. This was real. *Chris Mason was inside of that box.* I started to freak out.

Trying not to hyperventilate, I tried not to think of him lying in there dressed in a new suit, or maybe his Boy Scout uniform. But it came to me anyway. *He was in the dark!* This was no joke. He was gone. The beautiful boy who had so quietly, yet so vibrantly shared my life for such a short while was gone. As we exited the church, I watched Chris's parents and siblings take a left out of the breezeway, following the casket to the hearse. I wanted so desperately to go to the cemetery. I wanted to run after his mother and beg her to let me come with them. Instead, I continued to walk sedately behind my parents, heading toward the reception hall, all the while watching them as they lifted the casket and slid it into the hearse.

I had to get out of here. I knew I couldn't sit here at some reception with a bunch of strangers, sipping coffee and eating cake, waiting for Sue and her family to come back. I couldn't face her anyway. I had been a bad friend to her son. We drove back to Cornelius, mostly silent. I was engaged with my thoughts on exactly *how* I'd been a pathetic friend. After doing the math, I realized I'd met him almost exactly a year ago, yet I had to attend his funeral to know the basics. I'd talked about death right to his face. The memory of this conversation made me blush with shame. On Christmas morning I had pledged a few calls in the coming weeks, but I never dialed that number. I always got distracted by something—a party to go to, a friend to hang out with, or getting new clothes—and I'd catch myself making a mental note: *Don't forget to call him tomorrow.* But I always did.

How do you just plain *forget* a person?

That night, I went outside to try and clear my mind. It was cold and starting to snow. As I walked around the yard, I looked at the ground and then out into the darkness that enveloped our frozen fields. I looked at the ground again and felt the piercing cold of the night. Chris was in the ground. *They put him in the ground and now he's down there in the cold darkness.* I started to cry, and I stayed there, coatless, until I was done and my eyes were dry before retreating into the tiny, warm house.

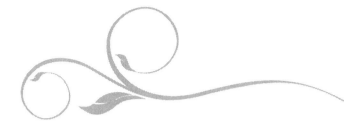

My life was a wreck. The approaching exams didn't help matters, but my test anxiety was derailed by my grief. I would cry periodically, every day, but I did an exceptional job of keeping it together in public. Every night I lay awake sobbing, sometimes for hours. Songs would set me off. Words would set me off. Half the time I could see Chris's ruddy face as if this day was no different from any day the year before. I was just going through the motions otherwise. Homework. Studying. Driving to school. Riding the bus home. All just memorized processes. I still went to mass every Friday at school, but only because I preferred it to study hall. For me, there was no God.

Not anymore.

One day, before exams, I was sitting in Hazel's class, blindly taking notes. I wasn't listening. I wasn't interacting. I wasn't functioning. He ended the lesson ten minutes early, instructing us to use this opportunity to study. Then he walked to the back of the classroom, which he never did. I stared down at my vocabulary sheet, not reading a word, feeling his gaze boring into the back of my head. What was he doing back there? I didn't want to risk a peek in case he was actually looking right at me. Was he about to give me a JUG for not participating in class? I really didn't need that right now.

The bell rang.

Thank you, *God*.

Everyone gathered up their bags and moved out of the classroom with the general clucking and flurry that befalls high schoolers. As I stood up to put my books in my bag, I heard Hazel say, "Lindsey." I paused. *Oh no*, I groaned inwardly. I turned around and looked at him. He waited, watching the rest of the students leave before he said anything else.

"I've noticed that you've stopped participating in class. You don't laugh anymore, either. Is there something wrong?"

I looked down at the floor suddenly confused, embarrassed, and feeling like I might snap, for good this time. If I did, I'd never get control over myself again. I couldn't look at him. I would start to cry if I did. How could I tell him what had happened? I couldn't. How could he possibly get it? He wouldn't. He'd be like all the rest and say, "Oh, I'm so sorry," or even worse, "I know how you feel." Excuse me? What are the odds that you know what it's like to survive cancer twice by fourteen, fumble your way into high school, and watch someone else succumb to leukemia just when you think everything will be OK? But most importantly, I couldn't let him see me cry. I tried my best to level my voice.

"Nope. No, nothing's wrong. I'm going to be late for class." The last thing I needed was a JUG for being late. I hightailed it outta there and zipped over to history. While I was blindly taking notes on the Ottoman Empire, Hazel went to see my counselor.

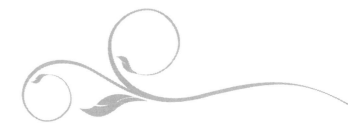

The next day, I received a note in class to see my counselor, Mrs. Forde. *Oh, great,* I thought. I wasn't interested in going to see just anyone and talk about this, but I didn't know who to ask for help. My first thought was Dr. Wolff, but then I realized that he was trained to deal with things like this all the time. How many kids had he had to watch die? No, Wolff couldn't fix it this time. I didn't think that my parents got it either. I couldn't bear the thought of trying to talk to anyone in Chris's family, though I desperately wanted to. I thought it would be insulting or make them suffer more than they must already. None of my friends at school had any real idea what I was going through. They tried to be supportive, but to no avail. Normally, everything they'd try to say produced the opposite effect of consolation. But if I went to a professional counselor, I was afraid that someone would label me as obsessive or depressed or something else. I didn't want to have to take antidepressants or see another doctor for the rest of my life.

I grudgingly went to Mrs. Forde's office. She was a very nice woman. I'd met her at Orientation. It was her first year at Jesuit, too, so I felt like we had at least one thing in common. She greeted me and showed me to her cramped corner of an office where I sat in a chair squeezed between her desk and the wall. "Sorry," she said. "You don't get a big office when you're new." I dropped my forty-pound backpack on the floor in front of me. She shut the door.

"So, Lindsey..." She walked to her desk (it only took two steps) and sat in the chair. "I've had a visit from Mr. Hazel. He seems to think that something might be going on. I think he's very concerned about you."

He narked on me! On the heels of that thought, I suddenly saw this whole situation from his perspective and was flooded with fresh guilt. Hazel was worried about me, and I'd been too selfish to be honest with him that, yes, something was definitely *going on.*

"He was telling me that, in the last few weeks, he's noticed you don't participate anymore like you used to, and he thinks you might be unhappy right now. Is there something that has been bothering you?" She looked at me inquisitively, but not expectantly.

I looked down at my bag on the floor. She wasn't pressuring me at all, which was great, but what could she possibly do? How would talking about it help at all? It wasn't as though she could change what had happened. Nothing could.

"You know," she said, "sometimes feelings can get pent up, and if we let them out, we can feel a lot better, and that's all it takes. But everything in this room stays in this room, and I won't make you say anything." She waited. I stared at the carpet. The clock ticked. I wouldn't be able to hold it in with this unbearable silence. How much should I tell her? We might be in here for hours if I told her everything.

Something snapped in my brain. I swear I actually felt a *pop*.

I told her everything. The whole story. From diagnosis to treatment to relapse to treatment to Chris's death to hating God, and then I told her about how I didn't have many friends and I was panicking under the stress of exams. With the first tear, she handed over a large box of Kleenex. I couldn't stop the tears; I had no handle on myself whatsoever. I wasn't even crying, I was *wailing*, and I would not be surprised if they could hear me in the classrooms down the hall. I cried so hard and for so long that I felt parched afterward, and so exhausted it felt cruel to have to endure class for the rest of the day. I'd been with Mrs. Forde through an entire fifty-five-minute period and we were well into another.

Mrs. Forde didn't offer any perspectives or suggest any psychiatrists. She just sat there and listened. When I'd had my last word, I sat there still looking at the floor.

She's going to tell your parents.

She didn't speak. Finally, I looked up at her. She said I could come back any time. When I left her office, though exhausted, I did feel very...blank. Even if it was temporary, I decided that this blankness was infinitely better than the unrelenting grief I had been feeling. I slept the whole night through for the first time in weeks. If I were still on treatment, I would have been at the clinic every week and either Dr. Wolff or Kaylee or Patsy probably would have noticed a problem long ago. I wonder now about what might have happened if Mr. Hazel had not blown the whistle on me to Mrs. Forde. How long would this have gone on? At least now I had admitted that I had this problem, and I had an outlet for healing.

Finals finally came and went. My grades that first semester weren't that great. I got a C in algebra, but surprisingly, I did all right in Hazel's class. When the report card came, PE was the first thing I saw. B+! How'd I manage that? The comment said, "Student gives best effort." Well, *yeah*.

I felt like I began to recover around Easter that year. While at the Good Friday liturgy, I had an epiphany. I'd been proclaiming all this time that God was dead to me, and I didn't understand how He could see fit to rip people like Chris from my life, never to return. But they told us in religion class all the time that He made horrible things happen to Jesus, and even though He was God, and Jesus was His only Son, those things had to occur for a greater purpose later—for the salvation of all humans everywhere. It dawned on me that perhaps my suffering would teach me something that would benefit others later. Perhaps much later, or perhaps I'd already helped someone else inadvertently. Then I realized I hadn't been a true atheist after all. I'd referenced God periodically over the last couple months, and if I thoroughly believed there was no God, then I wouldn't have continued to use His name. So there *must* be a God. Or at least, there wasn't *not* a God. Absence of evidence is not the same as evidence of absence. I could be open-minded.

The strange thing is that I never blamed God for what happened to me. He could've caused me to relapse a hundred times, and if I lived through them all, I honestly believe I wouldn't have had a crisis in faith. I blamed Him for what he did to someone else, which in turn, caused me to suffer the most profound pain in my life. What I felt in the months and years following Chris's death, and what I still feel today, is far worse than recovering from any surgery or enduring the malaise of chemo or testing. The physical pain always has an end, but the mental and emotional implications of what I'd been feeling were everlasting. Over time, they gradually faded, but there are always moments when they flare up as intensely and as painfully as that entire month of January 1995.

On the first day of the new semester, Hazel informed us that our semester project would be to present a poem to the class, and after reading it in front of the class, we would break it down stylistically and symbolically and dissect the lesson it was designed to teach. It wasn't bad. I didn't mind getting up in front of people and talking. After the bell rang, Hazel pulled me aside near the English offices.

"I have an idea for your poem, if you don't mind."

I shrugged at him. "OK."

"I think it would be brilliant for you to choose a poem that would relate to your experience as a cancer survivor. I think it could teach us all quite a bit." He looked at me, and I thought about it.

"You want me to read a poem and talk about how it relates to my life and how I've managed to...not die?" I asked him, almost unbelievingly.

"You certainly don't have to. Only if you're comfortable with it. It's something to think about, though." He ushered me out of the office and I headed to history, pondering his idea. Should I do it? I could. It wouldn't be hard. Yeah, OK. I could do that.

I chose a poem by Janet Lewis called "Remembered Morning." I'd never been into poetry at all, but I put myself into this one, try-ing to find any and all ways I could relate the text back to me. How's that for an assignment? You get up there and talk about yourself, which you're an expert on, for fifteen minutes, and you're done. Major points. I guessed I'd do pretty well if I did the assignment like he suggested.

Things were beginning to look up a little. I'd secured sponsorship for Dollie and me to compete on the Oregon Quarter Horse circuit for the 1995 season. Sharon arranged for Dollie to go to Sutherlin, Oregon, for training. She knew a couple who'd been working with youth competitors their whole careers, and they were very skilled and very positive people. So, Dollie left the farm in January and took the long trip south. This caused a problem for me, because I'd only be able to take lessons about once a month. In a way, the pressure was off because Dollie was taken care of and I could focus on school, but I really could have used some Wish Horse time during those difficult months after Chris had died. If there was a show in the Portland area, they would bring Dollie up so I could ride at the show, even if I wasn't competing. I longed for when I could make the trip for lessons. I'd spend the whole weekend down there, staying with the trainers and spending as much time on the horse during the day as was physically possible. Our first show was over Easter weekend, where I surprised even myself by taking second place out of ten or so. It was exactly the motivator I needed, and being around kids who shared the same passion for ponies as I was exactly the medicine I needed.

In the end, we had a successful season, considering that I'd never shown on that level before, and that we were only able to make it to three shows out of five that year. We took high point at one show, won a circuit at another show, and placed fifth in the state by season's end. That summer, I won my first 4-H medallion and qualified again for State 4-H, where we took blue in both classes. On the circuit, I felt like I was under immense pressure because while all the other kids had their parents with them, I was usually alone and was riding for the success that I knew my sponsor demanded. Despite all its frustrations and difficulty (and there were plenty—Dollie was not without an attitude, and neither was I), I was always happiest on the horse. Riding was the only thing I felt truly proficient at, and it was a unique skill.

In May, it was time for me to present Janet Lewis's poem "Remembered Morning" to my class.

I sat at my desk, listening to a couple other students give their presentations; then I calmly walked up to the front of the class. I wore a spring dress that day. I read the poem for the class just as Hazel taught us to read poetry—don't necessarily pause at the end of each line. After I finished, I set the poem down and picked up my outline so I could give my "lecture."

"This is a poem about significant memories. The most significant date of my life is November 9, 1991…" *That might be a lie, in light of recent events.* "…when I…" and it caught. The words caught right in my throat and I couldn't finish what I was saying. *When I was diagnosed with cancer. Just say it.* "When I was diagnosed with cancer." *Come on!* But if I wasn't careful, I was going to burst into tears again. My eyes widened in fear as the paralysis crept from my vocal cords over my whole body. God, why had I agreed to do this? What was I thinking? What had Hazel been thinking? As if I thought I was stable enough to be talking about this kind of stuff in front of twenty-five of my peers.

"…was diagnosed with pediatric kidney cancer." I had had to bite my tongue to keep my face from crinkling and losing it all together, but I kept plowing ahead. I rattled off my story, including the memorable day I met Chris, and when I was finished I came back to reality and took stock. No one in the class moved. Not even any blinks. I'm not sure anyone was breathing, really. Some kids had their mouths hanging open. I just stood there, awkwardly looking back at them, wondering if I could sit down now and how long this eternity would stretch out. Finally, Hazel started clapping, and my presentation came to an end the same way everyone else's did. I received 100% on that presentation. Good, at least the last three years had been worth *something*.

That summer was my last summer of freedom. I enjoyed working out at the gym with Mom, and I surprised myself by jogging two miles a day on the treadmill—to this day I have yet to break that record—and logging up to ten more miles a day on the bike. Perhaps that's not much by comparison to your average fourteen-year-old, but I felt as though I was in the best shape of my life. I was fit and trim–that leftover lung wasn't causing as much endurance trouble as I'd expected. The only thing that bothered me was my hair, which had come in almost black and corkscrewed. It looked like a huge fluffy helmet.

I continued showing Dollie and getting better all the time. At the local shows, we would clean house. At the circuit shows, we were improving consistently. We qualified for State again in 4-H, and took blues in both classes. I went back to camp for my second and final year as a camper. It would be four years until I could return as a counselor in training.

This whole time I had been completely without my periods—which was convenient. Then, partway through the summer, they returned. So, apparently I wasn't sterile after all.

Sophomore and junior years were infinitely better than my first year. I came to truly love being at Jesuit because it was such a tight knit, spiritual community. I finally knew my way around, I adapted to the workload, and I attended some retreats that really helped me ground myself in my faith. I had my small coterie that was made up of people from all the other "cliques," with friends from the choir group, drama group, athletic group, honor society group, and so on. Although I felt mostly at peace in this environment, I was looking forward to college, because Jesuit was, in a sense, a pressure cooker. They were always relentlessly pushing us to run faster, work smarter and be better, and that was hard sometimes. I knew though, that it was exactly what I needed to prepare me for my intended area of study. *Medicine.* I never had fallen out of love with it.

As time went on, I saw Dr. Wolff less frequently. Every month turned into every two months, then I'd only see him quarterly, then maybe three times a year, and finally biannually. Occasionally, it would be time for a CT or an ultrasound. I still had my port, just in case things took a turn for the worse again and for the convenience with blood tests, so I had to have Kaylee flush it out with heparin once a month. These monthly trips to the clinic were enjoyable. Quick and painless. It was fun to see everyone, and Dr. Wolff seemed to take some joy in seeing me well. After awhile, I wouldn't see Dr. Wolff in clinic anymore. The phrase, "What's your schedule next week? We should see you in clinic" to which I was so accustomed, gradually became, "What're you guys up to next week? Let's all have dinner." Dr. Wolff and his wife—also an occasional nurse of mine—gradually transformed from our caretakers to our social companions. I liked the social part, but after this went on for awhile, he began to suggest that it was time for me to see another practitioner for my long term follow up. I didn't like that at all. I hadn't been able to give up the Wolff security blanket. And I didn't want to. Plus, he started insisting that we call him Larry instead of Dr. Wolff. That just sounded weird.

Finally, in May of 1996, we'd reached the two-year anniversary of my last chemo treatment. I was cured. That was the day we ran the whole gamut of tests. Chest X-ray, CT, blood work, and I had to see the nephrologist, which also meant having a GFR. *Yuck*, I thought. *Nuclear testing. God, I hate that place.* Remembering my last experience, I felt ill. But it was no longer the canary yellow, cinderblock hell, and occasionally blood work can go without a hitch; and this was one of those times.

The results, however, were not typical. Dr. Wolff informed me that since my first GFR back in 1991, my kidney function had actually improved. It measured in the high ninetieth percentiles in all the GFR tests I'd had so far. What was remarkable about this test was that the function had dropped almost 50 percent.

"It's not how far it dropped that's the issue," Dr. Wolff informed us, "it's how fast it dropped that's of interest."

"So," I said, "does that mean that it'll keep going down?" I was afraid that my kidney would just crap out on me in a few years. I didn't want to think about dialysis at all. I'd seen pictures of what it does to you. I was *not* having them slice me open again to replace it, either.

"Well, GFRs can change continuously. If we tested you next week, we'd get a different reading," said Dr. Wolff. "How about you go down to Nephrology right now, and find out a little more." I walked over to Nephrology and checked in. When the doctor showed up, he had my GFR results in hand. He was an odd duck. He was very dull and a slow talker. "So, we've had a bit of a drop here," he said, eyeing the printout.

"Yeah," I said, nervously. *Duh, we've had a drop. We've had a freakin' cliff dive, doc.*

"The best way we can maintain your kidney is to alter your diet. This isn't a very seriously low function level we're talking about, but enough of a drop to need to be vigilant."

"OK," I said, waiting to see what I'd have to do for my "diet." He was thinking to himself for a while. Finally, he said, "I'd say low protein, low sodium, low phosphorus, and low potassium." I asked him what that meant. We discussed the implications. Low protein. Meat. Low sodium. No added salt or processed foods. Low phosphorus. Dairy products. Low potassium. Cantaloupes, bananas. Alcohol and high levels of caffeine should be out, too. Mom decided that I needed to see Sharon, who was a nutritionist, to go over a good dietary plan.

I took my diet very seriously. Everyone downplayed the severity of the issue, and that bothered me. Nephrology even said they didn't think it was necessary to ever do a GFR again, which I didn't understand. If my kidney was about to get worse, how could they ever know until it was too late? So, I took it upon myself to maintain everything to the nth degree. I took to drinking herbal tea instead of Starbucks mochas, which sucked because tea tastes like hot, bitter water to me.

Before I graduated from high school, Dr. Wolff sent me to his friend and colleague, an OB/GYN, to assess problems I was having with my menstrual cycles. Basically, I would have a full period for five days about every eight days. Sometimes it would go on for a while, or it might correct itself and then return months later. Because these problems were correcting themselves, the doctor didn't see any reason to do anything drastic or treat it with oral contraceptives. That was fine by me. The idea of having to admit that I took The Pill was too much for me to think about at that age. Plus, I just wanted to go about my life now that I was cured, and normal life didn't seem like it should involve taking meds every day.

"Now would be a good time to think about getting rid of that port," said Dr. Wolff with his typical shy grin. I felt strange when he said that. It had been there for so long now that I was loath to let it go. I knew it had to because a port isn't designed to be permanent. But what if they got rid of it and everything came back? That would suck, and in it would go again. I managed to hang on to my security blanket catheter for a few more months.

In July of '96, I said good-bye to my beloved port. It would be a day surgery, but they gave me a full-on general anesthesia, anyway. Holly came with us, and while we were on 14A, waiting to be called to the OR, we popped in a copy of *A Hard Day's Night*. For anyone who hasn't seen it, it's a black-and-white film where The Beatles run from scene to scene, singing songs. It was little more than primitive MTV. But as the movie played and the songs would come on, nurses would stop in the room to listen. At one point, as they played "And I Love Her," a small crowd of middle-aged women gathered at the door of my room. Everyone had a Beatles story it seemed. They took turns.

"Oh, my God! I saw them! When I was thirteen, I saw them! I was in Atlanta and I remember exactly how they looked! They wore gray, collarless suits with maroon trim...Oh, they were so beautiful..."

"Oh, yes! Yes! They were *so* beautiful! I saw them at the Coliseum in 1964..."

"Paul was my favorite," one sighed.

"Mine, too! Just look at those eyes," another agreed.

"Oh, look at him! He's such a showoff!"

"Have you seen the *Anthology*?" the oldest one asked.

"Omigod, are you kidding? How could I not?" another exclaimed.

While the ladies clucked and swooned at the Fab Four on the TV, Holly and I marveled at how we'd inadvertently attracted so much attention. Without warning, however, the crowd scattered when Transportation showed up with the gurney. I was off.

It was the usual routine. Go in to preop, sit for a while, go into the operating room, surrounded by masked strangers, breathe the gas, take a nap, and wake up. I'd only been out for thirty minutes or so. It was a really fast procedure. I woke up almost carefully, though. *A Hard Days Night* had distracted me on 14A, but in preop, I wondered and was afraid of how it would feel to come out of surgery. When I woke up, I felt like someone had scratched the hell out of my right chest. I felt the spot. The familiar round lump that I'd come to know and mindfully protect was gone. The scratch was the new incision that they carved right on top of the old one. I was puzzled. Why didn't this surgery hurt like the others? I asked Mom.

"They didn't cut any muscle this time. It's just like a scratch."

Oh. Yeah, made sense, I guess. I shifted in my bed, trying to sense a urine catheter. Nothing. Maybe I hadn't been under long enough. Or maybe they took it out in the operating room because it was only a day surgery. Who cares? At least I didn't have to deal with it. My biggest problem was coordinating myself to get to the bathroom. Even after short anesthesia, it's still challenging.

High school accelerated past me. Before I knew it, I was a senior. One of my teen dreams came true that spring when I was chosen as a member of the April Encounter team. I would, with eleven other seniors and a handful of faculty, lead forty-five junior men and women through a weekend spiritual retreat at the St. Benedict lodge on the McKenzie River. Right before I was scheduled to give my talk on finding love (and not taking it for granted), I was sitting on the bank watching the McKenzie roar past as the sun burned orange through the trees. It shouldn't come as a surprise that my talk on finding love was centered on Chris Mason, and as I sat there, chatting a little to God and talking to Chris as was customary for me anyway, I had a revelation: I have always believed that we fulfill a purpose in our lives. Our purpose may be grand or it may seem mediocre or we may not even realize we've done it and it trickles down and becomes significant later. But we all have one. At that instant, in the setting sun outside of Eugene, Oregon, in

April of 1998, I felt like I knew that Chris's purpose was to know me. To show me his life, and to show me his death. I knew that the reason he still haunted me in such a profound way was because I had yet to start executing my purpose. And my purpose was to be a physician and help other children and their families. To try and stop what happened to him and his family. This was as clear to me as the river running right past me. It all made perfect sense. I knew what I was going to do with my life.

Graduation came quickly. On that sunny, cloudless day, as I walked through campus draped in a cheap green gown made out of some petroleum product or another, and decorated with the telltale yellow nylon cords from the National Honor Society, topped with a green mortarboard and flopping yellow and green tassel, I looked at how much had changed since my first day as a freshman. Today's freshmen looked so small. I don't remember being that little. I didn't feel like I was as big and scary as those seniors I'd mistakenly met on my first day of school. A plaza now stood where once only a grass square had been, perfectly land-scaped and adorned with a super-sized bronze of the Madonna and Child. Where there was once an odd-shaped triangular build-ing and roundabout parking lot that passed as a theatre, now stood a multimillion-dollar performing arts complex complete with band, choir, and art classrooms; a black box theatre; and the main theatre—adorned with a baby Steinway. The campus had gotten a new coat of paint, awnings had been erected over the outdoor walkways, and all the buildings sported evidence of Jesuit's colors: green and gold. It was a beautiful place, and my memories of my time there were also beautiful. I took my diploma, glad to be done with the milestone of high school and anxious to make the best of my college years. I was going to be a doctor—just like the Wolff-man. The thought of it made me grin with excitement.

PART TWO: The AfterMath

The cancer experiences had been financially devastating. I don't know how they managed, but Mom and Dad scraped up enough cash to keep Travis and I in our schools. Because the financial consequences played out even years after I went into the second remission, there was talk in our family that college would not be an option if I couldn't get scholarships. I chose Gonzaga University in the end because their offer was the most fiscally sound decision out of all the colleges that had accepted me. It would cost less to go there than it had to attend Jesuit every year. Now that's a deal I couldn't pass up. I was excited to move to a different city in a state and region where I'd never lived before and knew nothing about.

I started my coursework in pre-med with the standard 100-level biology and chemistry and a ton of core classes: philosophy, English (which had *nothing* on Hazel's class), and visual arts. Pre-Med is certainly not without its challenges, and chemistry lab was my most difficult class, but I not only survived my first semester of pre-med, I did quite well, making the Dean's List.

But I was having problems with the competition. Of course, everyone and their dog is either a pre-med, pre-law, or engineering major to begin with. Quite a few of them drop out after a few weeks of academic overload and turn to business or history instead. In the end, it wasn't the academics that killed me; it was having to face the competition every day. A few girls who lived in my hall were not only brilliant in the classroom, they also somehow had time to do a ton of extracurricular stuff like row for the Gonzaga Crew or spike for Gonzaga Volleyball. They were beautiful and smooth. They probably still had all their God-given bits, too. I'd think, *How could I even have a chance getting into medical school when these people are applying, too?* So, by the end of my first semester I'd panicked under the scrutiny of my competition, dropped pre-med and much to my family's dismay, turned to broadcasting.

Despite the fact that broadcasting was dynamic and fun, there was something obviously missing, and this became clear quite quickly. An intellectual component that I had once gotten from chemistry, physics, and math was missing: a challenge. TV was more of a series of panic attacks and freak-outs about trying to get something on the air on time than it was the brain exercise in logistics. Now, TV had its own problem solving, but it was different than what I was used to. I still wanted pre-med. I kept my psychology major in hopes that it would remedy what I felt I was missing from TV. After all, it was a form of healthcare, right? Maybe I could counsel other kids who'd had cancer. That would be good. I could even be a doctor, still. But something about getting a PhD in psychology wasn't the same as getting an MD. I was still selling myself short. Psychology was definitely more challenging than broadcasting, but it still wasn't the grueling exercise in discipline and raw knowledge that I expected and desired. I tried to get myself on the fast track to becoming a medical reporter in TV news. That also was a process that would likely take ten years, and it made me think: if it was going to take that long and involve so much work anyway, why did I ever opt out of medical college? It was then that I realized I had made the wrong choice, and I was stuck with it. I'd chickened out and allowed my fear of failure to overthrow my sense of accomplishment. Oh, I was in trouble now.

I finished my degrees while working at a local ABC affiliate, where I completed a reporting/producing internship and learned the ropes of technical production. Immersing myself in TV news also brought to light the harsh reality of such a career choice. Long hours, low pay, working weekends, fast turnarounds between shifts—and forget about vacation and holidays. I learned that regardless of how much money you make and what market you make it to, job security doesn't exist. On the other hand, the disturbing gender gap that I'd studied in college did, in fact, exist. I would always see older male anchors with younger female anchors, and rarely, if ever, would I see the opposite. In fact, for the most part, older women were eliminated from talent positions all together. Did I want a job where my usefulness would cease the moment my smile lines turned to wrinkles? No, I wanted a job where I was appreciated for my intellectual accomplishments and acknowledged for contributions to my field. I decided that if I was going to work this hard, sacrifice weekends, holidays, and decent pay, I had better be enhancing the quality of life for at least one other person. In short, it seemed God was saying, *OK, you've had your fun. Now, I'm going to slowly nudge you back over in this direction over here, because you know that's where you belong anyway. Remember that day on the McKenzie? Come on, now.*

When I graduated in May of 2002, I decided it was time for a vacation. While the rest of my friends were jetting off to grad school, studying overseas, or hitting the corporate trail, I would take the summer to reevaluate myself and my direction in life. I was completely burned out from school and from working in TV news.

When you're going through the cancer process, love is about the last thing on your radar (unless, of course, Dr. Rainieri is in the room). What you care about is feeling well again, not whether or not you'll get asked to the winter formal. While sometimes it seemed silly to be thinking about how *dating* relates to surviving childhood cancer, it is actually an important part of re-acclimation into normal life. I cannot deny that it weighed heavily on me. In a lot of ways, this process was scarier than the cancer itself, because there were no clear directions. No protocols. I always wondered if normal girls my age made such a big deal out of learning how to date.

I was not a particularly popular girl in high school, though I was not invisible, either. I had my coterie, but let's just say I was never the life of the party, nor was I the frequent object of anybody's affections. In fact, a part of me still suspected that boys were infested with cooties.

All through high school, on some level, I simultaneously didn't care about and worried constantly about dating. I had all the same fears and expectations that every teenage girl has: when will I have my first kiss? What will it be like? Who will it be with? How can I hide this zit? How should I choose a boyfriend? Or should I wait for him to choose me? Do I have to meet his parents? Does he have to meet mine? Should I let him open doors for me? No, I can open doors for myself. Oh, God, it was endless. And dumb.

On top of these normal wonderings, I had my own special ones. What would boys think about me having survived cancer? Would it be an obstacle? Would boys be able to get past it? Would it weird them out? What I wanted was someone who could really appreciate the magnitude of the cancer experience and how it helped define me. But how could I get that when the memory of the confrontation with the college guys at Holly's house was still so acute? What about my scars? Oh God, was I supposed to be naked at some point? The days when I was nervous about being naked on an exam table were long behind me, but on a bed—that was a whole different ball game. My scars were in places not normally seen on a day-to-day basis, but there had been times where the incision line from my port would show above the neck of my shirt. And if I reached over my head, my shirt might reveal the long Tragic Magic Show in front. Both scars were still fairly red and noticeable. Inevitably, someone would pull me aside and subtly whisper, "Lindsey, there's a hickey on your boob …I just thought you'd want to know." Always in that hushed tone as if I'd been walking around with my skirt tucked into my nylons. At first, I was confused. I'd frown at them like they were crazy—because it started long before I'd ever even been kissed—and then it would dawn on me.

"Oh!" I'd say. "No, no, no. That's a scar from surgery. From the catheter that went *through my heart.*" It was my not-so-subtle code for *Stay the hell out of this.* And inevitably, they'd get this shocked look on their face and mumble, "Oh," and drop it. I'd look down at it and wonder how people could mistake a short, fat, flat line of scar tissue as a *hickey.* But then again, I didn't know much about hickeys to begin with.

Of course, I'd had crushes just like any other kid in high school. The guy I sat next to in keyboarding. A guy on the swim team. The lead in the school play. But I never had the self-esteem to make anything happen, and I was pretty sure the guys wouldn't come to me. Even though by sophomore year, I looked as healthy and deceptively normal as any of the other girls, I developed and accepted this idea that I might be considered "damaged goods" to boys. I knew that they knew what had happened to me. I settled for being friends with some and steering clear of most.

I am somewhat embarrassed to admit that Chris became the guy against whom I judged all other love interests and found them wanting. Crushes, friends, or boyfriends. In the brief time I had known Chris, he set the tone for all others to follow, though we never were even remotely "involved"–and I wouldn't have wanted to be back then. I still felt that our relationship quite literally "wasn't that way" in spirit. But I also felt that if a guy could measure up to Chris, then he would probably be worth my time. Slightly unrealistic expectations—these poor guys never stood a chance. The sad thing was, I looked for boys who would remind me of him. Eyes, hair, sense of humor, anything.

I did get my first kiss in high school. I thought that was pretty big accomplishment. I suppose everyone remembers their first kiss. Mine was not tremendously romantic. Because I lived almost twenty miles from Jesuit, nobody would come out to my house to pick me up. So I'd always meet the boyfriend at the Jesuit parking lot, and he'd always drop me off at my car there. The kiss happened when we were standing in between cars as I was unlocking my door. He went for it. There we were, standing in the Portland drizzle at eleven o'clock at night, in our high school's parking lot, under the harsh arc sodium glare of the streetlights, just kissing away. It was the most electric feeling I'd ever felt. It was also very wet.

Then about two or three months later, we got bored and broke up. I very much appreciated the simplicity of that process.

It was the only time it was ever simple. I dated three guys in college. Each one of them taught me some very specific lessons. I was terrified of dating in college because I'd heard about so many people who met their future spouse there. It felt so weird being at an age where we were officially old enough to be thinking about marriage and other major life decisions. Such decisions are a very normal process for normal people, but my appearance belied normalcy, and I was tired of making major life decisions. The concepts of marriage and children were complicated issues. It was one thing for a guy to think I might be hot and that we should go out, but whether or not I would be a good partner was something else. Again this idea of "damaged goods" came into play. Did guys want to marry girls who could have ongoing health issues? Did guys want to marry girls who would have trouble getting their own health insurance? Did guys want to marry girls who couldn't have children? Or rather, didn't *want* to have children? All the implications of my history were exhausting. And, oh, I was just so clumsy with love.

To say the least, I was naïve. I didn't understand the process because, like so many of my peers, I just hadn't had any practice. I was more worried than ever about my scars, and the worst thing

I could think of would be making out with some guy (oh my God, the naked thing again!) until he noticed the long slice across my stomach or the fat, curved line that wrapped around my ribcage and traveled up my back. I had a mental video about how he would handle it. He'd see it, freak out, make a comment about how ugly— or if it was particularly gross, "fugly" as the kids say these days—I was, and leave me alone and embarrassed. I cringed at the thought. The only way I could cope was to come up with humorous ways to describe the scars. I had a partner in crime in this, my best friend and roommate Sara, who'd had a small surgery on her shoulder. She found her scar repulsive, so we made a game out of it.

The place that marked the nephrectomy, once dubbed the "Train Tracks," became the "Tragic Magic Show." The title would inevitably elicit raised eyebrows, and I would describe being asked to volunteer for the "cutting in half" trick, and how it went horribly, horribly, *horribly* wrong. That the guy who did it was a hack and actually didn't know any magic *at all.* I'd also crack jokes about how if the black market kidney harvesters came after me, they'd open me up and find that someone had already beaten them to it. My port scar had come from a knife fight when I was valiantly defending my best friend from a mugger named "The Boss." Generally, I'd freak people out with the stories and they'd laugh and say, "No, way! That *happened?*" *Wow, I can't believe that worked.*

"No. Good story, though, huh?" It was a good icebreaker, at least. Somehow, it never turned people off that I was fabricating these elaborate lies–I think because the truth was harder to deal with.

The good thing about every one of the men I dated was that they all had the same response to my scars. They always said, "They're a part of you, and that means that they're just as beautiful." Maybe it was a line, but it worked to boost my self-esteem and gradually get over the whole "damaged goods" thing. After boyfriend #3, David, said it, I finally realized, *Hey, there's nothing to be embarrassed about here. This is who I am. God saw fit to create me with such a flaw that would leave me carved out like the proverbial jack-o-lantern, and that's it. I guess everyone has something, right?* Some people have depression. Some people are obese. And some people just live with the relics of trauma.

Despite the fact that the gents were understanding and accommodating of my physical appearance and the few restrictions that I lived with, it was tremendously difficult to find someone who truly appreciated what I'd lived through, and what I continued to live with. The thing about my cancers was that the experiences never really left me. It was something that was always present as a definition of me, like gender. *I'm a girl. I'm a cancer survivor.* Both had equal importance. And just like I saw the world through the context of being female (i.e., being disgusted by America's societal double standard for women's beauty), I also saw the world in the context of having survived a horrifying disease (i.e., seeing nothing but the terrible consequences that a smoking passer-by will face).

All three guys had been supportive to lesser or greater degrees, but no one truly understood. Tim didn't—he lacked the maturity and it always seemed to me that he used mild control as his coping mechanism. He always had to be touching me somehow, as if protecting me. He even declared to me once that he didn't like women because they were "irrational" and "high-maintenance." Though he said he liked me because I was very "logical and thought more like a guy." *Oh-kay.* Our relationship was a fun one for a long time. We learned a lot. We even discussed the idea of marriage, which I found equal parts exciting and nauseating. Then one day I woke up after ten months and instinctively knew it was over—I didn't want someone who would always try to be so "protective" of me. I didn't want a caretaker. My feelings were not precipitated by a fight or any other event; I just knew it. I think I pulverized his heart. It's not easy to do that to someone.

Then there was James. James didn't understand—he was too emotionally distant. I think that maybe he was afraid of my history, or intimidated by it, and he tried to use humor or a cool philosophical persona to cope. In his defense, I still think he was the funniest guy I have ever known, and I was laughing constantly. But I got frustrated quickly with the whole "Oh, well you know what Sartre/Kant/Descartes would say about that…" He had a great body, though, and I really gave it the old college try for a few months. Finally, I realized that when he went into philosophy mode (frequently), I just couldn't understand what he was *saying.* I broke it off. I didn't want a rationalist as a partner. I think I might have pulverized his heart, too. But this loss was different. I didn't grieve for it like I did with Tim.

Shortly thereafter I took a gamble and hooked up with a guy whom I thought might be—and even hoped—was The One. We had incredible chemistry. In a lot of ways we were very much alike. We laughed together nonstop. We had been friends for several years, and being with him was like being home—which made this relationship very risky to me. To my extreme sadness, I found out that David didn't understand me either, even though I most desperately craved his love and support. He didn't dare get close enough to even try. He was afraid, too, I think. Or maybe he just didn't care. Humor was his coping mechanism–not just with me, but with everything–and it aggravated the crap out of me. He was an expert at deflecting a fight, and so we never would actually accomplish anything to solidify our relationship. I wanted to leave him several times, but I believed in us and wanted him to love me. I thought if I stuck it out, if I was strong, we'd come out all right on the other end. What "other end" it was I envisioned, I don't know–this wasn't a scene in *The Shawshank Redemption*.

There was one other thing about him that doomed us probably from the get-go: David smoked. I didn't know at first and was appalled when I discovered it. From then on, I couldn't look at him any differently than I could at the smoking passers-by. When he finally plucked up the courage to admit he'd been in love with me for months, my first stunned thought was, *Nuh-uh!* And my second thought was, *Uh, but...you smoke.* Stupidly, I fell for the old promise: "Give me a month and I'll quit. *I promise.*" The worst thing about it is that I knew better. I *knew* that a month would become six weeks and six weeks would be six months and then it would never happen. And, of course, that's exactly what happened. Every time I saw him smoking or I smelled it on his clothes or his breath, or when I saw a carton of Marlboros on the shelf in his room, it broke my heart. The smoke and the idea of smoking and what it did to his body was enough to evoke flashbacks of my surgical recovery. All I could think of was what would happen to him twenty, thirty, forty years later. The thoracotomy. The chest tubes. The horrors of treatment. This all spiraled downward very fast. I became very depressed at the thought of it all. And I didn't know how to control these thoughts.

I tried to rationalize with him. I tried to help, but I just irritated him. I tried to tell him about what happened to me. Once I asked him, tearfully, "Do you know what it's like not to be able to breathe without excruciating pain?" He just looked at me, not saying anything. I continued, "I lost a lung and a kidney to cancer, and I didn't even *ask* for it." He shrugged, "Well, then, it doesn't matter whether I smoke or not. You didn't ask for it and you got it. So you shouldn't get so worked up about this." I flinched, as if he'd slapped me. I couldn't believe what he'd said. I stared at him, mouth agape, appalled. At that moment I knew it was over between us, though it was another few weeks before the relationship finally heaved its last death rattle. This experienced crystallized my feelings on the role of wellness in my partner—I couldn't be with someone who was constantly destroying himself.

Once David left, I started thinking that the only person who could ever appreciate life and wellness the way I did was another survivor. Then I feared that maybe the only one who could have really understood me had died in 1995. I missed Chris more now than ever.

That breakup was the straw the broke the camel's back, and it sent me spiraling into my third bout of what I would soon learn was post traumatic stress disorder.

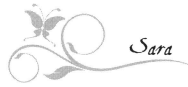

Lindsey has got a different perspective on cancer than most people do. For example, my mom is very dramatic about stuff, and about cancer she gets very quiet, whispering things like, "Oh, she's got cancer. She's a sur-vivor." *You know. Lindsey, however, was very matter-of-fact, like, "Oh, yeah, I had cancer, mmhmm." I think the first time we talked about it was not too long after we'd met in college, and she was mentioning camp, and I didn't know her all that well then. I said disbelievingly, "What, you still go* to camp *?" She explained that she was a counselor for a cancer camp, and she told me about how she was diagnosed and everything.*

Knowing about her cancer made me have a lot of respect for her. I thought, Oh, hey, there's more to this girl than meets the eye. *She'd had this crazy experience, and I just couldn't wrap my brain around what that must have been like—especially at the age that she was when she was diagnosed. Those were some bad years when she was eleven, twelve, and thirteen, especially when you compare that to what I was going through at eleven, twelve, and thirteen, which was more like, "Oh, someone just made fun of my hair," or "Ew, my nose is too big for my face." During those 'tween and teen years, girls can develop a lot of baggage—your personality is really starting to form; that's the time when eating disorders can become a problem and identity issues develop. But she had cancer instead! Little bit different experience than I had.*

It's the new term for what war veterans suffer from. But call it what you want. Whether it's shell shock or post-traumatic stress disorder, it's an incredibly grievous process. Mine was eight years latent.

The thing is, while you're a chemo kid, you're either too young to understand *really* what's going on, or you're too busy just living out the schedule and coping with all the vomiting to really think about it. When you come off treatment, you're so excited to be finished, all you care about is getting back to the life that every-one else around you has: eating whatever you want, exercising, breathing easily, *not* vomiting, etc., that you don't think about the what-ifs. In those days, there was no instruction manual for coping with not being sick. It sounds so silly that you need to be told how to be normal again, but it's true. They turn you loose on the world, saying you're "cured", and sometimes you can't handle it. I found that the further away from treatment I got, the more obsessed I'd become about potential long term problems and the harder it became to cope with memories. The thing was, while you're on treatment, the disease model becomes hard-wired into your brain, and there are all sorts of drugs to medicate any problems you're having. But when you're off treatment, no one is there to tell you how to cope with suddenly *not* having a disease, and you're left alone, struggling with how to deal and wondering if there are any other kids out there who feel the same way. There are. But I didn't know it then.

Since Chris's death, I'd had a number of small meltdowns. Nothing that interfered with my ability to function day-to-day, but I would find myself crying at night or fighting back tears in class, on the bus, driving my car. The breakdowns would happen periodically, generally during the holiday season, as I vigilantly kept anniversaries: his birthday, Christmas morning, the day he died, and the day they buried him. It was impossible for me to not keep the anniversaries. It felt insulting to both of us. Once, I even broke down in the middle of an all-school Mass at Jesuit that happened to occur on his birthday, and another girl from my choir had to walk me out of the gym to recoup. It was hugely embarrassing, having to walk out in front of the whole school, draped in the green and gold choir robes (which certainly didn't disguise me). But I kept things to myself for the most part. I didn't want to see a shrink or have to take Prozac. I didn't want to be another depression statistic. Depression was a fad at the time, and I was afraid I might be diagnosed even if I wasn't technically depressed.

After my freshman year at Gonzaga, I was undergoing an atypical trough—one so deep it seemed an abyss—and I finally snapped. I couldn't go on feeling like this. This was my first time with PTSD, and I knew I needed help. I went to Mom one morning and as we sat on the front porch in a couple of rattan chairs, I spilled my guts. I sobbed unceremoniously. I talked about how I'd been carrying this around with me for four-and-a-half years, and my troughs weren't getting better like I thought they would. I told her how the pain never dulled, and that there wasn't a day that went by without thoughts of Chris. I still carried a tremendous amount of guilt. I had bad dreams. I had phantom pains. The next day, Mom found a grief counselor, and I started therapy.

Vanessa White was a clinical social worker, and she determined right away that I didn't meet the classification of clinical depression, and that was a huge relief–I'd been terrified that I actually had a really big screw loose. I relaxed immediately. She taught me that grief never really leaves us but that it can dull over time, as our coping strategies improve. She posited that having moments of extreme grief is nothing to be ashamed of, and that it helps preserve the memory of someone with whom we were close. Grief over time is evidence of a bond. We discussed how Chris was real evidence of how close I'd come to dying, that he was the first experience I'd had with someone my own age dying. Of course it would affect me. She would be worried if it *didn't* affect me. Then she asked me if I had loved Chris. I said, of course, I had. Then she asked me if I had *really* loved him, and I said, "What? I don't know. What does that even *mean?*" She looked at me intently, the silence spinning out between us, and I understood what she meant. I hadn't really thought of that before, and, well, wasn't it all just a little too *convenient?* Too Hollywood? After all, I'd only been thirteen when I met the guy, and I hadn't had a romantic interest. Plus, it wasn't as though being near Chris had been all butterflies and electricity. After my initial shyness, it had been comfortable, simple, and just *normal.* It just *was.* And yet, all these years later, I was discovering that I was using him as a litmus test for other men.

"Oh my God, maybe you're on to something," I told her, "Maybe the reason I'm so hung up all these years later is because he was my..." Oh, I was embarrassed to say it out loud. "My first love?" I said, my eyes squinted a little. She nodded at me. I frowned, wondering about it, afraid of the idea. But maybe she had a point. There were other people in my life who had died. Family even. I was coping with all that just fine. And it's not like I was still devastated over Dr. Norman's death or anything. It took the whole summer, but over time, Vanessa helped me understand more about the guilt I had both as a survivor and as a lousy friend. She helped me define coping strategies for those days I would wake up feeling awful, the grief especially fresh in my mind.

There was no doubt about it. My heart had been wrung, and it had been broken. *Shattered.* But the resultant suffering was a mark of love, and it didn't matter to me whether it had been romantic not. Even though I had only known Chris for one year, it was a year better lived than if I hadn't known him; and if I had it to do over, I would not only choose the same but live it more thoroughly, more intensely. Basically, I would have done a hell of a lot better job on my end of the friendship. I felt that Chris played a part in God's grand scheme, and I play one, too, having known him. When I feel miserable about losing Chris, knowing that he'd never graduate high school, go to college, get a degree, have a career, marry the love of his life, or enjoy his own family, I try to remember that my life can be a tribute to him and all other kids who lost their battles. I realized, that someday, I will see him again. It might be tomorrow, it might be in one hundred years, but I will see him again. Chris Mason is not lost to me.

The trough that characterized the summer of 1999 eventually dissipated. Then, over the summer of 2000, I experienced a depression that I'd never had before. That was the summer that I was with David, whom I adored ardently but who seemed to, almost with all his might, pull away from me more each day. He wouldn't call, couldn't drive anywhere, would break dates consistently, and when we were together, he was somehow absent. I plunged into a depression, plagued with wondering, *What happened? What did I do?* I couldn't understand what was wrong with me. He kept saying he loved me. I was patient, understanding, and spent a lot of time, gasoline, and energy driving between the farm and the city to see him. It wasn't logical that he seemed so avoidant. That fall, as things deteriorated instead of improving like I expected they would, my nightmares started again. Then came the flashbacks and phantom pains. Certain foods, words, sounds, and smells could trigger them. It didn't help that David was a chronic smoker who'd broken a dozen promises to quit. I would cry often, and at a lot of things. I developed what I would later refer to as "tics." I don't know if they were actually textbook examples of tics, but I did have uncontrolled movement during flashbacks or phantom pains. I still do sometimes. They worsened for about a month, until I was hardly sleeping at all.

Then, much more abruptly than it all began, everything stopped. Later on in the spring, well after my symptoms had subsided, I took a class called psychopathology and found out that what I had been experiencing all these years had a name: posttraumatic stress disorder, or PTSD. It was a tremendous relief to know it wasn't just me.

I didn't seek help for the symptoms until a few years later, after I graduated from GU and moved to Seattle. I didn't think help was entirely necessary because the symptoms always went away on their own after a period of time. Sometimes they hung around for a few days, sometimes months. When I finally did get help, I found myself in the comfortable office of a clinical psychologist, warming myself in the sunshine streaming through the window and overlooking the yachts on Lake Union. Again, just like in grief counseling, I learned that there is no definitive way of curing PTSD, but that coping skills can improve over time and perhaps the traumatic experiences in question seem to move farther away. I didn't need drugs, the psychologist said, because I didn't meet the depression criteria. She suggested a hypnotist, just in case I wanted to explore that avenue, but I didn't. I'd studied a little hypnotism while pursuing my psych degree, and remembered the inverse correlation between level of education and success with hypnotism. Basically, if you don't believe in it, it probably won't work. I asked her about my "tics," and she cited a few studies that revealed some children on invasive treatments such as what I had for my cancers—especially those too young for verbal interaction—had been known to express their anxiety through certain motions in the hands, legs, and feet both during and after treatments. My movements were in my hands and arms, generally on the right side. She asked me what position I slept in at night. I explained that I was either a stomach-sleeper or on my back with my hands covering my abdomen. "You're trying to protect yourself," she said, smiling. Fascinating.

Those sessions didn't last as long as the grief counseling, and I learned little in the way of new techniques for combating my symptoms. The psychologist suggested meditation or yoga as well as keeping a journal to record the images and fears and get them out of my head. She said that having an active spiritual life helped cope with such trauma, and an exercise routine would help alleviate acute stress while priming the body to deal with long-term stressors. She suggested a few studies on long-term effects of survival and directed me to a few survivor's support groups. The thing that sucked most was that I did almost all of those things already.

"The important thing is to always remember that the frightening experiences are temporary and they *aren't real anymore*," she told me, "so keep that in perspective. Have a network of people you can talk to about these things; don't restrict your support group to one person. And always know you can come back here if you need to."

I left my last session feeling better but realizing that it would always be up to me. There was no operation or medication–no Wolff–that could just step in and fix this.

I still will hit my troughs and have bouts with the nightmares and the flashbacks. I spent a year on antidepressants that to my surprise and relief actually worked. Since then, I have learned that getting some sun every week keeps me off the antidepressants. The troughs happen less frequently now, because I am in a good place in life. They will worsen in frequency and intensity if I'm in an unhappy place in life—at a sucky, dead-end job or maybe going through a rough patch with friends or family—but I always seem to come back to baseline in the end.

Matt

The first I remember her talking about cancer was one night after work. There were three of us visiting, and she laid it out on the line. Everything. Almost like it was nothing. It was like she'd told the story a million times and it was no big deal. And I wasn't shocked by it like I thought I would be, because I really liked her. We were with another co-worker, Suzi, who was hearing this all for the first time, too, and she was totally floored. I remember Suzi telling me, "You can't go out with her! She had cancer! *What if she, like, dies on you?" I told her that had nothing to do with it.*

Her history, her memories of cancer, defined so much of who she is, but it wasn't the only thing about her. I saw how courageous she was. She brought a maturity to her young age that I had not seen before. I could tell she had grown up much earlier than most. And that's why our age difference worked out. In fact, she was too *mature for her age.*

I knew she kept a journal, and I respected that a lot. I was also really intrigued that she wrote it as if she were writing a letter to her friend that she had lost. Then after a while, I started feeling kind of jealous about this guy, Chris. In a weird way, it was almost like I was competing against him. But I also had a lot of respect for this someone I'd never even met, and never would. She would write such incredibly personal things to him, things that she wouldn't share with me *until much later.*

While I was enduring my life in Spokane–and that's really what it came to, enduring–two life-altering things happened. One, I met and developed a relationship with Matt, a photojournalist who worked at the news station with me. Two, I realized I was far overdue for a dental cleaning and checkup. I had to go find a guy in Spokane instead of my regular dentist at home, and I'll be forever thankful I did.

However, not at the moment I walked in to the office. When I walked in, I was more disconcerted. Someone was up on a ladder, working on stuff in the ceiling. There were ceiling panels lying everywhere, and a fine layer of construction dust coated the waiting room. Wires and cables were strung along the peripheries of the office. I was sent to an exam chair to wait for the dentist, when out of the corner of my eye, I saw the construction guy walk into a back room. A few seconds later, he reemerged in a white coat, sans the tool belt. He came over to my chair, sat down on one of those wheeled stools, and cheerfully said, "Sorry about the mess. Doing a little remodeling here, and installing a LAN." He reached for the long-handled mirror and scraper. As I opened my mouth, I thought, *Who knew MacGyver would be my dentist?* Should *MacGyver be my dentist?*

I'd never in my life known any dentist to perform a soft-tissue exam on the head, neck, and throat. He leaned the chair back and started feeling my head at the temples, down the sides of the face, along the jaw, down the neck and lastly, around the throat, near the thyroid. He was humming lightly as he did this and stopped when he got to my throat. After a few seconds, he said, "Swallow, please." He jabbed a couple fingers further into my throat and said, "Swallow again." I hate that feeling of pressure on the front of my throat, like it's blocking the windpipe. He paused a few more seconds. I waited, wondering what he was doing. Finally, he released my throat.

"I'm no specialist, but I do feel a small mass in your thyroid there."

I started to sweat. "What do you mean *a mass?*" I asked. This was the very last thing I expected to hear today.

He waved his hand. "Oh, it's probably nothing. I send about five patients every month to have things checked in their thyroid. Sometimes there are little cysts. They're no big deal. But you should go have it checked. Due diligence, you know."

My mind raced. Every time anyone had ever felt "a mass" on me, it had been *cancer*. On the other hand, my teeth were outstanding that day.

I raced home and called Dr. Wolff. He wasn't at the clinic. I called him at home, and rejoiced when I heard his terse voice answer. It was the happiest noise I'd ever heard. I started babbling at him. "Dr. Wolff, I went to the dentist today and he did a mandibular-esophageal exam and he said he felt a mass and he said I needed to have it looked at and that I might have a thyroid problem and that it happens all the time, and I had radiation to the chest and it might be cancer and I don't know what to do." I took a breath. I held it. Still kind of sweaty. The whole concept of having a mass in my body was awful. The concept of being a six-and-a-half-hour drive away from Dr. Wolff was just plain terrifying. The silence on the other end seemed to last for hours. *Why isn't he saying anything?*

Finally, he spoke. "Why don't you find an internist up there and have him or her take a peek at you." He sounded entirely unconcerned.

"Have I ever had problems with my thyroid?"

"Ah...no. No, your tests have always been in the normal range." I don't know how this guy could remember stuff like that off the top of his head but I thanked God that he could. He continued in a calm, somber tone, "Have them get some blood and run a TSH and a free T4. You can call me if you need to. I'll always take a call." I didn't know what a TSH or a free T4 were.

"Do you know any internists up here?" I asked him, desperately hoping he did.

"I don't, no," he replied. *Oh, crap.*

After I'd hung up, I wondered where I'd find an internist. Then I remembered the doctor who had treated me in the ER when I had a reaction to Septra antibiotics over the summer—full body rash, really fun stuff. He'd recommended someone, so I looked him up in the yellow pages.

"Dr. Henkle is not taking any new patients," droned a bored female voice.

"You don't understand," I insisted, "I've been *referred* to Dr. Henkle by the ER at Sacred Heart."

"I'm *sorry*," the voice insisted back, "Dr. Henkle isn't taking any new patients."

God, why can't I catch a break? "Well, then," I said, gritting my teeth, starting to get angry, "does Dr. Henkle have any colleagues who *are* taking new patients?"

"Male or female?"

"I don't *care*." Somewhere inside I registered that this woman was doing her job and trying to be considerate, but, God, people! My very life was at stake!

"And what is this regarding?"

"I have a mass in my thyroid," I said brightly. I should have said *I probably have cancer for third time.* It might've gotten me in to someone sooner. But she seemed not to care.

"I can get you in to Dr. Hu, but she doesn't have an opening for a week." *A whole week?* My God in heaven. Spokane sucked. If I'd been in Portland, the Wolff-man would have had me in tomorrow morning. That is a distinct benefit to cancer care: it can get you to the front of the line a lot.

"No one has any openings before then?"

"No."

OK, now I was pissed. Now I had to *feed* this thing for a week before anybody cared to look at it.

"Fine," I said, indignant. It would all be fine. It had to be. Right?

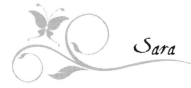

Sara

It's funny. Lindsey's cancer-dentist was a really good dentist. He was a total MacGyver. I have been to a lot of dentists, and I cannot find one anywhere who gives a crap about my neck. But when she first told me what he had found, I thought, "Eh, it's probably nothin'."

It made me remember that from the moment I met her back in our sophomore year of college, she was crazy anti-smoking. She hated cigarettes. Hated them. *It wasn't until she found out about the thyroid cancer that I finally figured out why she hated them so much. I was always like,* Oh, yeah, sure, smoking gives you cancer. *And here I was sucking on these sticks that the carton* says *gives you cancer, and then suddenly my best friend had cancer. I thought,* Hmm, maybe I should put these down.

Matt

When she'd been to the dentist and she was getting scared, I tried to downplay it all to help her feel better and keep from panicking. My role was "Let's not worry about this until we know there is actually something wrong with you. There's no reason to worry before we know that there is something wrong. So let the doctors do their things and we'll cross that bridge when we get there." I hoped that would give her a little comfort, but it didn't. Not very much, anyway.

I figured I'd better let Matt in on what was happening. I liked the guy. He was older but didn't look it. We met when I had just turned 20, and were both working at KXLY-TV. I thought he was twenty-five. I found out later that he was thirty. That gave me some pause, but really, I enjoyed spending time with him. And after my most recent devastating failure of a relationship, all I wanted to do was have some fun. And Matt *equalled* fun—even when we were on the clock at the news station, racing down the Spokane streets to a story, radio blasting Everclear, singing at the top of our lungs. After we had been together for about nine months, he took a job in Seattle, and so we were doing the Long Distance Relationship Thing, which I was leery about. But I was hopeful because the best part about him was that he was 100 percent a Good Decision Maker, and that's the type of person I could make a life with. I thought he would really be able to Get It. As I dialed his number, I thought, *Well, I'll find out now if he does.*

When I told him what the dentist had found, he was not responsive.

"Huh, interesting."

I was speechless. Did I even *know* this man anymore? He'd only been gone a few weeks and was already alien to me.

"Wait," I said indignantly, "I tell you I have an unknown mass in an area that just happened to endure radiation therapy ten years ago and all you can say is '*Huh, interesting*?'"

A pause on the other end. "Well, you don't know anything about it yet. Why worry?"

Now I was pissed. I had thought once upon a time that this man might *Get It.* Boy, was I wrong.

"Why can't you just appreciate the kind of psychological trauma this means for me and be supportive? Can't you understand what kind of memories this elicits?" I was livid.

"Because it isn't *anything.* Not yet, and it probably won't be." He was clueless. I couldn't talk to him anymore. I was dumbfounded that he could be so *dumb.* I felt the hot sting in my nose and throat that said I was about to cry, so I ended the conversation and cried myself to sleep.

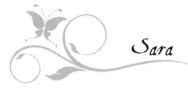

Sara

I don't know how much time passed between the dentist visit and the confirmed information. I don't think she said anything to me at first. When the information finally came out, it was like, "Oh, my God, how can this be happening? This is just not real." Her cancer diagnosis really changed the way that I saw the world. Other than really old people I'd known in my life, she was the first personal encounter I'd had with cancer. Especially someone who was my age. Cancer wasn't anything that had ever crossed my mind as a remote possibility.

Now, I think differently. Now we're all getting a little older and we interact with older people, and so I think about it more.

On the tenth of February, I sat in the waiting room of a clinic on the South Hill in Spokane. It was the oldest medical building I'd ever been in. It had that old building smell, mixed with the telltale clinic reek—that amalgamation of rubber, alcohol, and hand cleanser—and it made me very uncomfortable. I dreaded this entire day. I knew there would be a blood draw, and that it wouldn't be pretty. It never was. I was that girl that phlebotomists and nurses dreaded. More importantly, I didn't know what this mass was, and I didn't want anyone but Dr. Wolff to look at it. I tried to distract myself with thoughts of Matt's scheduled visit that weekend, but I was still kind of angry with him.

They called me in. I sat on the butcher paper and gave the ten-minute schpiel about my medical history to the medical assistant, provided Wolff's clinic number, described how my dentist had felt a mass, and waited impatiently for Dr. Hu to show herself. I tried not to think about all the possibilities. When Dr. Hu finally arrived, I was surprised to see she showed no trace of Asian heritage— she looked more Norwegian than anything. I wondered in what other cultures the name "Hu" could possibly originate before I thought, *You stupid. She married into the name.* Honestly, sometimes my mental torpor even surprises *me.* She examined me: BP, pulse, temperature, heart, breathing, etc. *Finally* she started to feel the place where the dentist claimed he felt a mass. It was about freakin' time.

"Hmm…I don't feel anything." She dug her fingers in harder. "No, I don't feel anything." I looked at her like she was crazy. Did this woman pass her Boards? "Are you sure he said it was on the right side?"

"*Yes.*" I did everything in my power to keep from exploding at that point. How had I managed to pick the one doctor in Spokane who couldn't palpate the thyroid properly? I wanted Wolff there more than ever. In my current state, no one but Wolff would do, no matter how good they were.

Dr. Hu couldn't feel anything, so she ordered an ultrasound for the next day, and the blood work. I went to the lab and proceeded to thoroughly embarrass myself via hyperventilation, shaking, and tears for the next few hours as they tried to get blood out of me. I wished for Kaylee or Patsy. I reflected that out of the hundreds of blood draws I'd had in my life, only one ever went perfectly. It was well into my remission years and a day during which Kaylee, Patsy and Dr. Wolff had tried and failed multiple times to get blood. Wolff finally tossed his hands up and said, "Come back tomorrow. And bring some wine." So I did. Kaylee poured an ounce into a sterile urine cup, and instructed me to drink it quickly. We waited a bit until I could feel the heat setting in. Then Wolff examined my arm and exclaimed, "Firehoses!" It was an easy and instantaneous draw. If only we could have figured that one out years ago. If only I'd remembered to bring wine to *this* blood draw. God bless those nurses, though. They were soothing and made me feel as comfortable as was possible–which was next to impossible to do. In the end, it took four people. One to do the draw, one to hold the arm still, one to wrench my head in the other direction, and the other to hold down the rest of me. When it was all over, they brought me chocolates and some cold water in a sterile urine cup. I wrote the entire lab a thank-you card the next day. I hope some people got a bonus or a raise because of it. They certainly deserved one for dealing with the likes of me.

That night, the places where they'd needled me turned into enormous green and purple bruises with bloody looking centers. Matt arrived at about midnight, saw my arm, and said, "Huh, interesting." I clenched my fists. Yeah, I was still mad at him for acting like a soulless freak, and he wasn't exactly helping himself with that response.

I went for the ultrasound a few days later and, drawing upon previous ultrasound experiences, expected the technician to provide comment if he found anything interesting. He didn't say a word the whole time, and I lay there with my throat covered in the clear, cold goo, dozing in the dark, listening to the hum of the machine. When the test finished, he cleaned off my neck and left. When he came back to give me the OK to go, I thought, *Well, it must have been a fluke, or he would have said* something. *Maybe I owe Matt an apology.* I went home and went about my day without another thought of it, and a relief that perhaps I *had* made more of it than was necessary. I didn't expect a call for two days, per the sonographer's advice.

Dr. Hu called that evening.

It's never good when they call earlier than they say they will.

"Lindsey, your TSH and free T4 levels were totally fine."

I sighed with relief, saying, "I didn't expect them to be off. I've always had normal function. I don't even have any symptoms." So it was going to be all right, after all. Score one for Matt.

"Yeah," she trailed as though reading a checklist, "so that's good. But on your ultrasound…" I felt the bottom drop out of my stomach, and terror gripped my chest. My heart raced at breakneck speed with an intensity that almost hurt. "…there is a 1.8-centimeter mass with calcifications on the right horn of the thyroid."

"Calcifications…" I mumbled.

"Yes, calcifications…sometimes that can mean malignancy…" She drifted off.

"I know," I breathed. I sat there for a second, thinking that every nightmare I'd had in the last eight years had just come true. I came back to life for a second. "What now?" I asked. I was in a daze.

"Now, we need to do a fine needle biopsy to be sure whether it's malignant or something else." She started to say that she'd make an appointment for me when I interrupted her.

"Um, I'm going to call my oncologist in Portland. I'll call you tomorrow."

"OK."

I sat on the edge of my bed, cross-legged, not knowing what to do. Then, like a wrecking ball, every memory I'd ever had about cancer and treatment slammed into me. I started to cry. I didn't know whom to call. Mom? Matt? Dr. Wolff? Probably all three. Well, maybe not Matt. But I felt paralyzed. Images flashed in my mind: lying in the hospital bed, walking for the first time after surgery, pulling out clumps of my own hair, vomiting, vomiting, vomiting. I held my tears in. When you live with six other college kids in a cheap rental house, it's hard to keep secrets. And I didn't want to talk to anyone about this yet.

Someone knocked on my bedroom door. Sara. She saw me and said, "Oh my God!" she shouted. "What happened?" Sara had been my best friend since we met when we shared a dorm suite during sophomore year, but I still couldn't be totally free about what was happening. Not even to her. I was a train wreck inside but as stoic as an Easter Island head on the outside.

"They found something." My voice was all high-pitched and awkward. Then I stopped. I needed Dr. Wolff. I ran upstairs to find his number in the address book. I dialed him at home. Voicemail. Damn. I called Mom. She answered the phone and I started to cry.

"Lindsey, what's wrong?" she demanded.

"They found something. On the ultrasound."

"Listen, Booie, have you talked to Dr. Wolff?"

"No, I can't reach him."

"Everything is going to be fine, OK? We need to get a hold of him first." Mom and I finished our conversation and clicked off. Almost instantly, the phone rang. I answered it.

"Lindsey."

Relief. Oh, praise God, Laudate Dominum, Halle-*lu*-ia, I knew that voice! "Dr. Wolff!" I shouted, and heaved a sigh of relief.

His clipped tones were soothing. He continued, "Please. Please. Call me *Larry*. We just walked in the door from San Diego and saw you on the caller ID."

What marvelous luck–I was actually catching that break I'd been after. I told him what had happened, ending with, "The internist says she wants a fine needle biopsy next, but I wanted to talk to you first."

He was quiet on the other end, contemplating, before saying, "Yeah, I think I'd prefer that one of my colleagues take a look at you. When can you get here?" he asked.

I looked at my watch. Today was Wednesday, February 13. "Uh, I can get on a plane tomorrow."

"I'll see you in the clinic at eight a.m. on Friday morning. Bring your labs. And the ultrasound if you can get it."

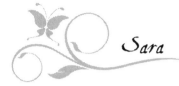

Sara

I cried to our big-brother/roommate Pike Meterson (a jumbled version of the letters of his real name that was, for reasons not well understood by the rest of us, the name he preferred that we call him) about it all when Lindsey had gone back to Oregon. I don't think he cried, though. Pretty sure not, actually. Then I had to have all these conversations during class with people I didn't know very well. Because she was gone all the time, people started asking me questions. I tried to be delicate, saying, "Oh, you know, she's at home. She's sick right now." And they would ask with what, and I'd say, "Um, with cancer." They would proceed to freak out big time, and I was like, well, what am I supposed to say? It was all very stressful. And no one could tell me how to deal.

There were a million things to do between the time I talked to Dr. Wolff and the time I was supposed to be on a plane. I started by calling Mom back and informing her that Dr. Wolff requested I be evaluated at Doernbecher. Then I got online and purchased a flight to Portland on Southwest Airlines. One way. We didn't know for sure when I'd be coming back, or, worst-case scenario, *if* I would be coming back. I called Mom back with the departure and arrival times. She said she would clear her schedule to meet me at the airport. I felt better now that I'd had an initial catharsis and that I was completely task-oriented. I always do better when I have a plan. I called Matt that night and told him everything. He was, as usual, mostly unconcerned. Absorbed in his new job, he mentioned that he was leaving for Arizona in two days to cover the Seattle Mariners at spring training.

I was aghast.

"What, you're leaving for *Arizona?*" I stuttered indignantly.

"Well, yeah," he said as if I didn't hear him the first time. That made me angry.

"Still?" I squeaked.

"*Yeah,*" he said, calmly yet obviously.

"Uh, even though I have to go do all this stuff at the hospital?"

"Of course," he said in the same tone. That only made me angrier.

"Why?" I asked, feeling the heat burning in my nose and throat. The floodgates were threatening to burst again. They would if he wasn't careful.

"What, do you expect me to leave my job when we don't even know what you have, *if* you have anything at all? I can't just *not* go to Arizona. It's *Spring Training*. And besides, this is my new *job*."

That was the moment. Right there. I lost all respect for the entire world of sports, and TV. I couldn't believe what I was hearing. Could he have *been* any less there for me? I started to cry but did my best to keep him from hearing. I couldn't stand the idea of him knowing he'd made me cry. I hated him at that moment.

"Do you have any idea what this is like for me? Any idea?" I demanded. He didn't respond. "Do you know that this is the nightmare that I have had repeatedly for the last eight years and it's coming true?" Still no response. "Do you know the horrific things going through my mind right now?" I challenged him, "And do you remember the conversation that we had last summer, about how if it ever came back, I don't want to go through all of that mess a third time? Bone marrow transplant! *That's what they would do!*" It was getting too hard to talk. I got off the phone as fast as I could. While I packed my suitcase, I wallowed in my terror, confusion, and fury.

The thing was, I knew how it would come out.

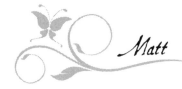

Matt

I'd convinced myself that the cancer was totally in the past and it couldn't come back again. I just felt like it was history. Even when she found out about the thyroid cancer, I was like, "Oh, it's all right. You probably just picked up some extra radiation from before. It's not a big deal." I had learned it was a common cancer in women and that it's very easy to cure. So I just took the mindset that everything would be fine. I don't think she appreciated that.

I was just trying to be comforting, rather than understand how she felt. Before she knew she got the thyroid cancer, I was still taking the positive approach, saying, "Listen, they have to be extra careful, so let's not worry about it until we need to." And that was why I chose to go to Arizona.

I slept fitfully that night. The morning of Thursday, February 14, dawned beautiful, mild, and sunny. I raced through the dodgy end of Spokane's downtown, looking for the medical records library. When I found it, I ran in, and they handed over a big envelope labeled with "ULTRASOUND" in huge block letters.

"These are due back in one month," the lady said flatly. She really looked like she enjoyed her job. *Fat chance*, I thought. *I paid for these, and they're pictures of* my *giblets. I'm not returning them.* Afterward, I raced up to the South Hill, picked up my labs, and jetted back to the house. I had enough time to scarf down a mediocre lunch and haul my suitcase upstairs. Sara volunteered to drop me at the airport. As I was piling my stuff by the back door, getting ready to leave, the front doorbell rang. I ran across the kitchen and living room to open it. A guy was standing on the porch with a clipboard.

"I have a delivery for Lindsey VanDyke?" he said.

"Yep. Right here."

"OK, hang on a sec," he said as he hopped off the porch. I pulled the drapes aside and saw a florist van parked on the street. Of course, it was stupid Valentine's Day. He brought back a vase crammed full of two-dozen long-stem, blood red roses. I thanked him and closed the door. I walked back to the kitchen and put them on the small round table in the corner. There was a tiny box of truffles in the roses, and a mini envelope. I tore out the card and read it.

Sara walked in and started jumping around and cheering, excited that I'd gotten flowers. Pretty soon, all the other girls in the house came in, attracted by Sara's commotion like bugs to a light. They lauded me, saying how lucky I was to get such beautiful flowers and how great Matt was. They all sniffed and smelled them. They all read the card. They didn't know what an ass he could be on the phone when you had cancer.

"Too bad I don't even get to enjoy them," I shrugged. "I gotta go." They all looked simultaneously crestfallen. They all knew I was leaving, but I think more than one had forgotten where I was going and why. "Happy Valentine's Day, guys," I said, trying to be cheerful as I gestured toward my flowers. They said they'd take really good care of them while I was gone, so they'd still be alive when I got back. I didn't bother mentioning I didn't know how long I'd be gone. Sara said, "Take one with you!" She pulled one out, wrapped it in wet paper towels, and wrapped that in foil and finally a little plastic bag. It did make me feel a little better, but I didn't think it would last the flight. I held the flower as I rode to airport in Sara's pickup truck, with my films in my lap. I wondered just what the hell was going to go down the next day.

Of course, airport security required that I X-ray my flower and my ultrasound, which of course, meant they got smashed up. I almost had it out with one of the security officials for crumpling and wrinkling the films, but decided I didn't need to be detained anywhere, that I was maxed out already, and I bit my tongue.

On the plane, the closer Portland got, the more anxious I became. I knew I wouldn't be able to sit still until they could tell me exactly what this little mass was. While I was lost in my thoughts, the woman sitting next to me asked if the ultrasound was mine.

"Yeah, it's mine." I tried to keep my voice even, calm, and pleasant.

"Oh!" she exclaimed, delighted. "Are you having a baby?" I wrinkled my nose. *No way, lady.* I looked down at envelope, wondering which would be worse: being pregnant or having cancer again. What should I say? If I lied and said yes, she'd want to talk about babies with me. I'd have to tell her.

"Uh, no," I said, still looking down. "This has pictures of what might be cancer. I'm going to Doernbecher to find out." She seized my left hand and held it through the rest of the flight. We talked about Doernbecher and how great the new facilities are. I told her about the cancer I'd had already, and how much I respected and adored my oncologist. We talked about what might be on the ultrasound films. Then, with my rose and the envelope resting on my lap, she reached over and took hold of my other hand and started to pray for me. Out loud. She even got the woman sitting next to her to pray, too. I kind of looked around with my eyes because I could feel everyone else in eyeshot watching, but I didn't care. Hers was the most touching, genuine response to my situation yet, and I was thankful for it. I tried desperately not to cry, but despite my best efforts, fat tears rolled out of the corners of my eyes.

When I walked out of the airport, I'd regained control of myself. I saw Mom's cherry red Yukon pull up with Sandy Dunes, tail wagging, ears pricked, tongue lolling, and wearing a purple neckerchief, in the back window.

The next morning, Mom and I walked into the Pediatric Hematology/Oncology Clinic at Doernbecher Children's Hospital. Dr. Wolff was standing at the nurses' desk, writing notes in someone's file. He wore dark Dockers, a short-sleeved soft yellow oxford, and a red bow tie. He directed us into a room for a moment to talk. He'd arranged for me to see a colleague in the Pediatric Endocrinology Department, Dr. Estes. Dr. Estes was a major brain when it came to tumors in the thyroid. I found it funny I was still seeing pediatricians. Truth be told, though, I preferred them to the grown-up docs. Wolff explained that because of the nature of thyroid cancer, if that was what we were dealing with, he didn't treat it and I would need to see someone else. "Why?" I asked him, surprised. I didn't like the idea of being treated by someone else.

"Thyroid cancer is so mild it's almost not considered a cancer, so we aren't very adept at treating it up here," he said. I'd never thought of that before. The moment I'd heard cancer was a possibility, I'd assumed that this would be the exact scenario for which we'd so carefully prepared back in 1994 with the marrow harvest. It would be another Wilms, and I would be having a marrow transplant. I said as much to Dr. Wolff. He said no, thyroid cancer would not deem a marrow transplant. Befuddled, I went with Mom to Peds Endocrinology. Dr. Wolff shouted for us to stop back in the hem/onc clinic before leaving that day.

Dr. Estes was a young-looking man, who'd agreed to see us before he opened for the regular clinic hours. I got the impression it was a favor for Wolff. It's nice to have friends in high places. Later on, I heard Mom say something about Dr. Estes's new patient waiting list being nearly nine months long. I sat on the butcher paper and watched him look at the films and the labs.

"Well, there it is. Little guy about 1.8 centimeters," he said. Then he turned to the labs. "Your thyroid function is completely normal. Have you had any symptoms?"

I thought for a second. I was vaguely familiar with symptoms of hyper- or hypothyroidism. "No, last fall I lost a bunch of hair, but nothing since then."

"OK." He came at me with his fingertips. I held still, though I loathed the feeling of being prodded on my throat. He "hmm"ed through the exam as he tried to locate the mass. Finally, he jabbed a few fingers as far into my throat as he could, and his face changed.

"There it is," he said, sounding half-relieved. "Boy, it's really in there. It's incredible that your dentist found that." I posited that maybe it was because of the angle at which I reclined in the dentist's chair. He nodded, "That's a very good point; I'd believe that." He went to call his colleague, a head and neck surgeon, to have a look. When he came back, he was almost excited, saying,

"This is very unusual, but we have a group of fellows down here for the day, and it would be excellent if you'd be willing to let them have a look at this thing. It's in a very unique place, and we're impressed that it's already been found. Would you mind if they came in to examine you?"

I didn't even have to think about it. I waved my hand at him. "Do you know how many of those kids I've put through this institution over the past ten years? Send 'em in!"

Dr. Estes left to get the fellows, but came back alone, ushering us out of the office to go to Head and Neck Surgery so I could see a Dr. Rogers. Too bad for those fellows.

The exam chair in Rogers's office looked like a hybrid between a dentist's chair and an electric chair. When he came in, the first thing I noticed was his bow tie. I love the doctors with the bow ties. He had a prominent jaw, and there was a light strapped to his forehead, kind of like what a spelunker might wear, which I found hilarious. I restrained my laughter, however. After we talked about what was going on, he proceeded to assemble a little fiber-optic doohickey, saying, "We're going to have a look at your vocal cords with this. If you can hold still, it'll just be a few seconds."

He started to snake the line down my throat, and I gagged. "All right, we've got a great gag-reflex there. That's great!" He really was genuinely pleased by my gag reflex. He switched on some kind of motor and attached this little spray head to a hose and said, "How about some anesthesia? This stuff tastes a bit like an old tire, but it'll work." He squirted the fluid against the back of my throat. It burned slightly and it did taste like an old tire. We sat there for a second, waiting for it to work, and he asked me what I was doing with college and what I wanted to do for a career. I told him I was on the cusp of graduating, working in TV and going to take the summer off. Then he slid the fiber-optic line down my throat again, and then pulled it out. "Vocal cords look good," he said. He did a perfunctory exam and felt for the mass, which he located immediately. I was impressed. He sat down in a chair.

"The next step will be to do a fine needle biopsy." The word *biopsy* set me off. Needles in my throat, and ones long enough to reach whatever was lurking way up in there. I could see him talking but wasn't really registering what he was saying. "...smallest needles available. Generally, there's no need for anesthesia." I wondered if lidocaine would be enough. "...probably do it Monday, if possible," Dr. Rogers finished.

I shrugged. *Whatever, people. I'm just along for the ride.* But, nothing drastic was going to happen that day, and I could look forward to a whole weekend of sitting on pins and needles. Dr. Rogers got me in for the biopsy on Tuesday morning at eight a.m.

We stopped in at the hem/onc clinic to brief Wolff.

"We saw Dr. Rogers and now we're scheduled for the fine needle biopsy on Tuesday," I said.

"Oh, yes, yes, yes. Dr. Rogers! He's good." Dr. Wolff nodded approvingly, arms crossed. Apparently Wolff and Rogers were chums. He thought for a second, head down, arms still folded across his chest as was typical for him. Finally he said, "Tuesday what time?"

"Eight o'clock in the morning."

"Anesthesia?" he asked. I glanced at Mom and shrugged.

"Uh, he said they generally don't use it."

Dr. Wolff suddenly was overcome with a comical look and almost snorted derisively as he half-laughed, half-ordered me to contact anesthesia and make sure they were there to knock me out if necessary.

"I'm thinking it will be in their best interest," he said, leaning slightly toward me while raising his giant eyebrows and grinning. He always got a lot of lines in his forehead when he did that. Oh,

God, he was absolutely right. He sent me home that day with a script for diazepam (a benzodiazepine used for antianxiety), too. Just in case. The Wolff-man knew me better than I did.

The weekend passed. Thankfully, Mom kept me very busy. The only times I started getting upset was at night when I was by myself, trying to sleep. When I managed to sleep, I was haunted by horrific dreams about giant spiders. Classic Jungian archetypal symbols. The common theme among them all was that the spiders would bite me, which would cause a lot of uncontrollable pain, they would continuously grow, and I could not kill them. If I managed to kill one, another immediately appeared in its place and started to grow. I would wake up, uncomfortably sticky from sweating. The fact that Matt was in Arizona instead of with me (where he was *supposed* to be, I didn't care if he was the President of the Freakin' US of A) didn't make things any easier. Monday night I lay awake and sobbed the entire night away. Maybe I should've taken one of those diazepams. When I heard my parents get up at five thirty a.m., I thought, *Oh, the hell with it,* and got up, too. Today was the day.

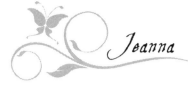

Jeanna

It's easy to forget how wonderful a phone call without attached tragedy can be. You always seem to get bad news from phone calls.

Matt

I didn't know how intense a biopsy was, putting a needle into her throat. I thought it was just some test they would do. That was my first mistake. My second mistake was thinking that since she had her mom with her, it'd all be fine. Maybe I would just get in the way. The third thing I didn't understand was that all of this was probably streaming back a lot of memories for her, making it difficult, opening a lot of old wounds from ten years before; and none of that stuff even crossed my mind, mainly because I'd never had to go through anything like that.

I guess I was the one who was immature.

Jeanna came with us that morning. The waiting room was packed. They were overbooked. In the hall, far from all the other patients, was a very obviously ill prison inmate. He was in a wheelchair, wearing the telltale orange jumpsuit, and was little more than skin and bones. Two police officers escorted him, one on either side. They just sat out there in the hall, the prisoner staring at the floor. I pitied him. Maybe he committed murder or something else equally horrible, or maybe he just had a lot of parking tickets. But he was human and obviously suffering. Once I looked up from my book to see that one of the officers was holding a trash can so he could vomit into it. I wanted to talk to him and find out what he had and if it was cancer. But I was afraid, not of what he could do to me—he was obviously not capable of much—but of the principle of talking with an inmate. The other people in the waiting room would stare at me. So much for being a good Christian.

Finally, it was my turn. Only one adult was allowed in the room with me. A doctor with what sounded like an Australian accent came in (Mom later laughed at me and said, no, he had a speech disorder—but it sounded foreign and sexy as hell to me) and started the procedure.

"Wait, where's the anesthesia?" I asked.

"There's no anesthesia ordered on your chart," he said.

"No, we called on Friday," I retorted. He shrugged back at me.

"Well, they're not here. Do you want to do this tomorrow instead?" he asked.

I thought hard. No, I couldn't handle another night like last night. I wanted to know what was in me now. I tried to be rational. How hard could it be? They said they hardly ever used anesthesia anyway. I could probably do it. Just have to buck up and be a man.

"No, I want to get this done." It wasn't comfortable, even sans the needles. He had an ultrasound wand he was pressing all over the place. God, I hated the feeling of someone pressing on my throat. I have been known to get weirded out if my turtlenecks were too tight. My neck was stretched out and my head tilted back as far as I could hold it.

"Hmmm…it looks like it's hiding right behind the jugular," he said, tapping keys on the machine. "But that's OK." He looked at me and a smile barely touched the corners of his mouth. "We'll get it. We'll just have to dig a little more." Dig? *Dig?* I couldn't see what he was doing. I didn't like not being able to see. I'm a control freak. Then I felt a pinch and I jumped.

"Just the lidocaine," he cooed. "We use just a topical anesthetic to dull the needles going through the skin." I lay there, tense, waiting for him to withdraw the needle. Then I thought, *What about all the tissue under the skin? Will that hurt?* While he prepped the needles and waited for the lidocaine to work, I started getting wiggy. Then I saw the first needle. Oh yeah, it was thin. At least as thin as a butterfly, but Holy God it had to be eight inches long. He came at me with it. I pushed away, reflexively. He came closer. I edged farther away, stifling my sobs.

"Lindsey, I need you to hold still, here," he said quietly. Mom turned my head toward her and held it in place, but that only made things worse. I started to shake, and I couldn't hold in the sobs anymore. My breathing had become irregular and too fast. They tried to calm me down. I was able to get a hold of myself and slow my breathing. They tried again. Again, I started freaking out. The idea of someone rummaging around in my throat with a super long needle was too much to wrap my brain around. I started hyperventilating and shaking again. It was so embarrassing.

The needle went in.

I didn't feel it enter.

But I sure felt it underneath the skin.

I did my best to hold as still as I could. You'd think if you were as tense as I was, you'd be able to hold stock still. Not so much. I'd try and hold my breath to keep from sobbing, but then I'd take a big, hitching breath, and throw the needle off course. He'd pull it out and try again. Then he'd leave the room so I could calm down, come back, and start over. God only knows how long I was in there. The second time he left the room, Mom grabbed my face with both hands and tried to "tough love" me into cooperation.

"You need to get a grip! You're an adult now!"

I zoned her out. I couldn't believe what I was hearing. How was insulting me going to calm me down? "Leave me alone! Do you have any idea what this is like? Do you want to try instead? If you're going to be like this then you can leave!" I hissed back at her. She clammed up. The doctor came back for a third pass. I was determined to make it this time. I was able to keep from sobbing out loud, and I kept the shaking to a minimum, but it was the hitching breath that got me.

"It's very close, we're almost there, OK? I need you to hold completely still for me."

OK. I tightened up and held my breath. *Go, doc, hurry.* He wasn't hurrying. *Hurry, dude, I gotta breathe. Go, go, go, go.* And before I knew what'd happened, I'd hitched a wet, sobbing breath and blew the whole thing. Exasperated, he pulled the needle out and leaned forward, resting his elbows on his knees.

"We can't do this. Not today," he said sternly, pulling off his gloves. "You're going to have to come back tomorrow, and I'll get you anesthesia." I started to cry hard. And very loudly. We'd gone through all that for nothing! It felt like we'd been in there for hours. The mattress on the gurney was literally wet from me sweating so hard. My neck and hair were coated in iodine, and they'd gotten me with the needle at least three times and it was all for naught? He wrote orders for anesthesia. "Make an appointment with the desk for tomorrow morning. Don't eat anything after midnight. Come in. The nurse will start an IV and will be here for the whole procedure." He left. Mom calmed me down and we walked out of the hospital. I was mortified.

Driving home, I sat in silence, thinking. I'd just been to hell itself this morning. That was, without a doubt, the worst procedure I had ever been through. All I could think of was how Matt was cheating me, hiding behind his stupid job in sunny Arizona, watching baseball, so he didn't have to be here for it. The whole experience still brings tears to my eyes.

Linda

That biopsy was pretty nerve wracking. They did so many needle aspirations! Were they using her as a pincushion because this was a medical school? It took hours. I didn't understand why it had to be so difficult.

There was, again, a lot of speculation and anxiety about this biopsy. When Dr. Rogers started to explain the details and the prognoses, we started to feel better. He said that there shouldn't be any problem with it. This was a common cancer, and even if it should come back, we could just do the nuclear ablation again. It was like, "OK. I can deal with this."

Matt

I never considered that she'd refuse treatment. First of all, Linda would totally kick her ass. I knew, though, that once she realized how small of an ordeal it would be she'd choose treatment.

The next morning, as my stomach growled loudly for all to hear, we started over. I laid on the gurney with the pillow under my neck, stretching it out. A cheerful, middle-aged woman came in, saying, "Good morning! I'm your anesthesia nurse today!" I liked her immediately. She described the types of drugs I would get: a benzodiazepine to start, followed by phenobarbital. I would feel dopey and sleepy but would be able to communicate completely and follow directions.

Of course, she couldn't find a vein. For an hour, she fought with both arms, hands, and even feet, trying to find something, anything to access. Every try failed. After about four tries, I was, as usual, embarrassed and a complete emotional wreck. Why did I have to be like this? How was it that Dad could have big soft veins like fire hoses running under his arms, and I had these all-but-impenetrable coffee stir-sticks? After the fourth go, she gave up and left the room. She returned with a small syringe.

"Let's try an oral benzodiazepine and see if that doesn't relax you so we can get in." We were already late. I always wondered what the docs and nurses thought when they ran across patients like me. Was I a complete and total inconvenience? Dr. Wolff seemed to always take it in stride. But these strangers hadn't known me for the last eleven years. I put it out of my mind. The last thing I needed working me up was the obtuse concept that I was a scheduling inconvenience. I squirted the syringe in my throat and swallowed it. We waited. Next thing I knew, the nurse announced, "We're in!" I looked down at my left wrist. We certainly were.

The same doctor from the day before came in and prepped my neck with iodine, then fired up the old ultrasound. "Here comes the phenobarbital," the nurse declared. "Take a hold of my hand and squeeze it if you need more, when you start feeling things." The procedure felt a lot like the marrow biopsy Dr. Stein did years before. I'd feel pressure and moderate discomfort, and I'd try to move away from it. Someone would say, "Hold still," and I would. No crying. No hitching breaths. No embarrassment.

Next thing I remember is Mom putting my shirt back on me. Then I remember riding out to the car in a wheelchair, and then someone putting a seatbelt on me. Once, I heard that the true definition of anesthesia is that which induces paralysis and amnesia— I certainly had spotty amnesia. Later Mom told me I had eaten lunch and even had a few conversations–which I don't remember. I don't remember getting into the wheelchair or the car, or getting out of the car at home.

They pierced the tumor with eight separate needles that day.

Dr. Rogers said pathology could take up to forty-eight hours, and that he would call as soon as they knew. I knew what it would be but nonetheless desperately hoped mine were false intuitions. Mom said that the samples had been full of blood, and that the doctor had mentioned that blood generally signified malignancy. It didn't look like a good day for false intuition. When I'd slept off the last of the anesthetic, I looked at my neck in the mirror. Eight little red holes decorated the area around my collarbone. It hurt.

One night, as we were racing Sandy Dunes around the house after a dog treat, the phone rang. I picked it up, still laughing at how such a chubby pooch could move so fast.

"Lindsey, it's Dr. Rogers." Buzzkill. Docs don't call for fun, and they don't generally call at night if there's good news.

"Hi, Dr. Rogers," I said flatly. Mom, Dad, and Travis stopped and waited. Sandy Dunes chewed and then coughed on her Pupperoni.

"It appears the tumor is in fact malignant. It's what we call papillary thyroid cancer…"

The verdict was in. The jury had spoken. I had been right all along.

"…good cancer because the cure rate is so high. It's very non aggressive, and your tumor was caught incredibly early." Even though I'd been expecting it all along, I still felt shocked. He continued, "So, you don't have to do anything right away. Thyroid cancer is incredibly slow growing. We could wait until after you graduate—"

I interrupted him. "No. I don't want anything growing in there. Every time I eat, I'll feed it, and I just can't handle that."

"OK, that's fine. We'll be scheduling surgery in the next two weeks."

"OK," I said. As I hung up, everyone was looking expectantly at me. "It's cancer," I announced, tossing up my hands a little.

Mom demanded the details, which I gave her. Then she said, "Well, you better start calling people," and sighed. As if it was something *I'd* done wrong and I needed to take responsibility for. I frowned and started going through the list of who I'd call: roommates, grandparents, Matt.

I decided to call Matt first. I'd talked to him briefly already that evening. There was no answer on his personal cell. I paged him. No answer. I tried the news car's phone. No answer. I tried the sports department phone. No answer. I tried the assignment desk at the station, so I could try and get his hotel number. Nobody knew where he was staying. They transferred me to the sports anchor. By this time I was almost in tears, completely worked up over the fact that the one person who I thought was supposed to be here in the first place was now completely unavailable and a thousand miles away. Eric, the sports anchor gave me another number, which I dialed hastily.

"Hello?" It wasn't Matt's voice. I hesitated for a second. It must be the reporter's phone.

"Hi…I'm looking for Matt?"

"Oh, sure. Hang on." It was loud in the background, like they were at a restaurant or something. Finally, I heard his voice.

"Why did you turn off your cell phone? Dr. Rogers called."

"Oh, yeah? What'd he say?" Matt asked, unconcernedly. He was snacking on something. I could hear it crunch.

"It's cancer," I said bluntly. I waited. I didn't care about his reaction. I was so spent after trying to track him down, and angry that he'd left me alone to go through all this that I hoped he started sobbing right there in public. He didn't.

"It's cancer?" he asked. The tone was totally different.

"Yeah. Cancer. Papillary Thyroid Cancer."

Suddenly, things got quieter on the other end of the phone. "OK, I'm in another room, now, where it's quieter. So what else did they say?"

"I'll have surgery in the next couple weeks, and then they'll talk about treating it."

"OK." I could hear some concern creeping into his voice.

"So…are you coming back then?" I asked.

"Yeah. I'll make some calls tonight and see how soon I can get there."

That night, while trying to sleep, I thought about what had happened. It felt very surreal that my worst nightmare had come true. *It's not fair.* When I went into remission in 1994, I always made decisions that would prevent my returning to the hospital. I ate well. I exercised. I didn't smoke or do drugs. I hardly ever drank. And yet, here I was with cancer again. Chemo. Radiation. Side effects. Vomiting. Surgery. *Marrow transplant.* God, I didn't want any of those things. I'd said as much to myself. Now God, if one existed, was calling my bluff.

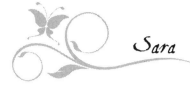

Sara

When I got the call I was super worried. I remember crying about it for sure, thinking, Oh, this is not a good thing. Not good. *I didn't know what to say to Lindsey, because obviously there is nothing to say in that situation that would make anything better. I didn't want to say, "Oh, it'll all be OK,"because, well, maybe it* wouldn't be OK! *I didn't know what to expect. Would they put her on chemo and stuff again? Would she be able to finish school? I also started to look at how I lived my life and examined the kinds of things that I did. What was healthy? What wasn't healthy? How healthily did I want to live my life? Suddenly, I became very aware. She was my friend, my age, and just like me. And if it was happening to her, it sure could happen to me.*

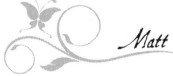

Matt

It suddenly became real when I got that phone call in Arizona. I was in total denial that any of this could be a problem, that it could ever be cancer. I was never even worried. When she called, she was so upset, and that was upsetting to me. She was angry at me, and I felt bad then. It brought to light everything I had denied to that point. I was in Arizona with a co-worker, and we talked about it that night. Then I had a lot of time to think when I was on the plane to Oregon. When I got there, I went into Full Support Mode. I have a pretty level head, so even if something like cancer comes along, I don't overreact to it. I don't freak out about it. I deal with it in a businesslike manner. I'd probably do exactly the same thing if it happened to me. It's just how I am.

Jeanna

I hadn't heard before, that once you'd had cancer you're predisposed to get it again. Again, one of those little things in the fine print that they didn't tell me about!

I returned to Gonzaga for about a week or so before surgery. I met with all my professors and my advisors to discuss my academic plan for the last semester of my college career. The Communications Department arranged for some course substitutions, a drop and double count that reduced my course load to twelve credits. My professors agreed that I could take whatever time I needed to recuperate and that we could work together so I could graduate on time. I had to write chapter summaries for any seminar sessions I missed. So I was still on track to graduate on May 10. Now I just had to get this pesky cancer thing out of the way.

I wasn't in a good mood. Having to discuss the issue at hand with multiple people all day was very depressing. Then I had to arrange my absences through the university, which meant that the priest who headed up that particular department wanted to counsel me. The whole thing was overwhelming, and still, I wasn't sure I even wanted to be treated for this. Images of chemo and flashbacks of side effects played on a permanent, endless loop in my brain. In between meetings, I collapsed into a chair at a corner table in the Crosby Student Center and tried to hide behind a *Gonzaga Bulletin.*

Unsuccessfully.

"Hey, Linds, how's it goin'?" I knew that voice.

David.

How did he know it was me? I thought I'd managed to conceal myself well behind the newspaper. I plastered a fake smile on my face and lowered the paper. He sat right down at the table without even *asking* if he could join me. I started to fidget. I really didn't want to talk to anyone right now, much less an ex. That's what I get for resting in the Student Center, I suppose.

"Nothin' much," I droned flatly. I was having one of those dual-personality moments like you see on TV where the character is behaving outwardly in a very calm and predictable way, but internally they're fantasizing about throttling the other person. I decided that I'd just clam up as much as possible, hope he'd take a hint and leave me be. I looked him straight in the eye the whole time. In retrospect, I should've just asked him straightforwardly to leave.

"Hey, guys, what's going on?"

Ex #1 walked up to the table. Tim. I was besieged! "Lindsey, how are you?" he said, a little too casually. I wanted them both to leave. Now. So I answered his question truthfully.

"My life is shit."

He cocked his head at me, confused. "OK…"

He turned to David, and they discussed a class they had together. I looked hard at my newspaper, pretending to read but just really staring at the words. Then he left. One down, one to go. I looked back at David. He looked back at me, a little warily as he leaned forward a little.

"Linds, what's going on?" He asked in in a genuinely concerned tone. Bless his heart. He wasn't *trying* to antagonize me. I looked down at the table in shame and to try and get control of the tears I could feel collecting in my eyes.

"I was diagnosed with cancer. Again." I looked back at him. All I could think about was the scene in *Forrest Gump* when Tom Hanks says, "…and so I went. Again. And I met the President of the United States. *Again*…" Except that meeting the President would actually be cool. This was just going to suck. David turned white, and his face fell.

"Oh, Lindsey…oh, Lindsey…*oh, Lindsey*." Now *he* looked about ready to cry. I wished he'd stop saying that. I continued to stare at him, desperate to prevent myself from shedding a tear. He blundered through the usual "I'm so sorry" and "don't worry, you can beat this," euphemisms, which I couldn't stand to hear anymore. How could people presume to think what I could and could not beat? That just because I'd done it before meant that I would, could, or even *wanted* to do it again. I hated how everyone could be so damned positive, so *insistent* about the concept of battling and beating cancer, when all I could think of was how it would feel to go through it all again. The average person has no idea what it is really like. They read about celebrities' bouts with cancer, they see that they've beaten it, and they internalize that everyone can beat it. But until you've actually participated in the process in some way, you know nothing.

"Is there anything I can do?" he offered. A small voice in me rejoiced, *He still loves you!* A larger voice in me snorted derisively.

Now he wanted to be there for me? Where was he eighteen months ago?

"No." I crossed my arms and shrugged. "There's nothing. Except...you could make me laugh."

He tried desperately and lamely to crack a few jokes.

"That didn't work," I said acutely. We eked out a few more minutes of awkward conversation before I finally had to get out of there, or I'd go crazy. I felt these days that I could go crazy at any second and that *actually* throttling someone wasn't such an outrageous idea. "Well, I gotta run. I have all sorts of things to get in order before I leave again."

"Oh, OK. Well, see ya, Linds."

After everything was over, and I had a few seconds to myself, I admit I handled the encounter with Tim and David the wrong way–but especially with David. I let my anxiety turn to rage turn to shameful spite. This would prove not to be the first time I would act out during this cancer process, but nothing that had happened between us in the past would mean he had somehow earned this from me.

When she went in to surgery, it was hard for me. I hated to have to see her go through that. When they wheeled her away, I was a little bit of a mess. Her parents were there with me, so I knew everything would be OK. Sure enough, before we even knew it, we found out it all went fine and she was in recovery. Once we could see her, I never left her side until we were headed home. I was holding her hand after surgery. Lindsey didn't even know it for at least three hours, but it impressed her mom. I stayed overnight when the rest of the family went home, even though the nurses tried to chase me out after "visiting hours" were over. I slept on the floor for a while until they figured out I wasn't going anywhere and brought me a chair to sleep on.

March 7 at 6:30 a.m. I walked into the admitting lobby of Oregon Health and Science University with Mom, Dad, Jeanna, and Matt in tow to begin the all-too-familiar surgery process. With the bracelet wrapped around my wrist, I walked down into preop and was directed to a bed. I changed into the telltale magenta, backless gown with snaps down the sleeves. Just like old times.

Mom was with me, but everyone else had to stay in the waiting room. After a while, she said, "How 'bout I go get Matt?" While she was gone the nurse came in to start my IV. Matt came in and tried to keep things under control. It was the usual travesty. Several needles and a couple extra people to hold me down later, they got in and I relaxed completely. A team of surgeons came through eventually.

"You ready to go?" one asked.

"Sure. I have the easy job: take a nap. You guys have to *work*."

"All right, then. Let's go!"

Matt kissed my cheek. They rolled my bed through the double doors and into the operating room. Again.

I woke up, feeling dopey, and the front of my neck felt irritated. I touched it. There was a large plastic dressing covering everything from my collarbone to my jaw line. Everything hurt. I felt nausea.

I'd never felt nausea after any other anesthesia I'd had before. I felt like I couldn't breathe, my nose was running, and I was about to throw up. There was an oxygen line under my nose. I'd always hated those things, blowing cold air into your nostrils. I pulled it out, actually feeling like I could breathe better that way, and tried to sit up. God, I was a wreck. I was in a large, open room with a number of other patients. Recovery. Some people were starting to move around. Others still looked dead to this world. A very large man in the far corner started thrashing around as he was waking up, and all the nurses rushed over to him.

I was gonna puke. I needed a barf bucket, pronto!

"Wait," I croaked. I tried to yell, but all I could do was whisper. "Help." Nobody heard me. No one came. Fine. They weren't going to pay attention to me, then I'd just vomit all over myself and the bed and they could deal with it. A nurse finally came over and gently pushed me back down on the bed, replacing the oxygen tube and admonishing me to keep it in and to stay down. I went back to sleep.

A hand wrapped around mine. I turned my head to the right and felt searing pain at my throat. Tears pushed out my eyelids. Matt was standing over me. He brushed my hair back off my forehead. I dozed. Then Mom's face replaced Matt's. I slept again.

I woke up in my room. It was a double, and we didn't have the window bed. Mom, Dad, Jeanna, and Matt were all clustered around the bed, watching TV and reading the paper. Matt had his left pinky wrapped around my right. I still felt as though I couldn't talk. Everything ached. I still felt a little pukey. But at least I was in a bed and not on that hard gurney. Mom started telling me about how I'd been in recovery for a really long time and Matt muscled his way past the nurses to get in and see me. Nobody argued with him or put up a fight. The guy was 6'2" and 265 pounds, stacked like a body builder. She told me that the surgery went very well. The parathyroid glands were closely attached but not embedded in the thyroid, so Dr. Rogers was able to get me out of the OR ahead of schedule. But while in recovery, they realized there was no bed for me on the ward, so I had to stay down there until one opened up. After Matt initially got past the nurses, they all took turns sitting with me, one at a time.

"It was really scary," Matt said, "seeing you like that. Your eyes were rolling in your head, and your tongue was hanging out. You kept trying to take out your oxygen line and move around. I almost started to cry. I'd never seen you like that." I was touched. Maybe he finally *Got It* now.

Every four hours someone would come in and take my vitals. Blood pressure, temperature. Just like old times. I actually felt very at home. Similarly, every four hours—not on the same schedule as the vitals, of course; that would be too easy—a phlebotomist would come through to do a draw. They were checking my calcium levels. The parathyroids are responsible for calcium regulation. When they are disturbed, as is the case with this surgery, calcium levels in the body can plummet. Rogers wouldn't discharge me until the calcium levels were back in the normal range. My nurse would bring me a paper cup of fruit-flavored Tums to chew on. The last time I'd had Tums was long before I'd ever been diagnosed with the Wilms. Much to my surprise, however, they were quite a tasty dish.

When I woke up the first time, I felt something squeezing my lower legs. Squeeze. Release. Squeeze. Release. It was irritating. Looking down, I noticed there were two balloon-like wraps Velcroed around my legs. They were attached to air hoses and a pump that would regularly inflate and deflate them. I couldn't sleep, and I wanted to desperately.

"Can you take them off?" I asked the nurse. He slowly shook his head at me.

"We can't take them off until you start walking for us. They are keeping the blood from pooling in your legs and clotting." *Oh. I suppose that's all right, then.* But I could do without the "fffffffft!-shshshshsh" of the pump. Why had I never had anything like this before?

I could tell by the layout of the room and the hallway outside that I was in the old South Hospital wing. Surely I was on 8, six floors below my old haunts on 14A, which was nowadays a maternity ward—or so the rumors went. The new Doernbecher Children's Hospital opened in the summer of 1997. I'd helped build that hospital with my work on the Holiday Cards for Kids campaigns, and here I was stuck in the old South hospital. There's irony for you.

I knew then that being a kid and being in the hospital was much more fun than being an adult in the hospital. Here, there were no colors on the walls, no one to come around and do magic tricks, and the staff had no sense of humor whatsoever. I'd try to crack jokes to lighten the mood, or to at least make myself feel better. No response. Well, occasionally a "hmm." Thank God I'd had cancer when I was a kid. Compared to *this* it had almost been fun.

My hair was crusty with topical iodine. I felt the skin around my huge plastic dressing. It felt like leather. Matt said it was red and blistered. Great, I had a giant red, leathery bib. Mom posited that I must have reacted to the iodine. I agreed, though I'd never reacted to topical iodine before. I'd used it often back in the days of the Neupogen shots, and Kaylee would prep my port with it for an access. Curious.

Dinner came that night, and I almost automatically ordered them to send it away, out of habit. But I was hungry. It hurt to swallow, that much I knew from the Tums. I hoped it was soup. That would hit the spot. Jeanna lifted the plastic lid and revealed a brown lump surrounded by mashed potatoes and corn. Mmm, boy. "What is *that?*" I whispered. Silently, we all stared at it. Finally, Mom started laughing.

"I don't know what it is!" she exclaimed. Jeanna took the order form out from under the plate.

"London Broil," she read flatly. Then, with wrinkled nose and furrowed brow, she added, "Why, of all things, would they give you *London Broil?*" I picked at it, ate some corn, the Jell-O and, of course, the ice cream. We sent the London Broil itself back to the kitchen, untouched. Well, at least they were still crankin' out terrific crap for food here. Some things never change. To this day I have never understood how the cruise industry makes so much money feeding thousands of people fabulous meals at least three times a day, while hospitals can't seem to ever tempt anyone's palate. And the price of a hospital room per night is about the same as the presidential suite on a ship. Maybe the hospitals should hire cruise industry executives to run the show.

Anesthesia wreaks havoc on your sleep schedule. Suddenly you're dozing all day and awake all night. I was bored all night. Again, Matt had asserted himself and against nurse's wishes was staying overnight. But there was no place for him to sleep. So he tried in vain to sleep on the dirty, cold linoleum floor using his coat for a pillow, I was thankful he stayed. Not because I felt he deserved to be here, going through this with me for once, but because I found his presence calming. He was, somehow, normalizing. Eventually I dozed again but awoke early in the morning. There was no clock, so I tried to guess the time based on the light and activity levels in the hall. Yep, those students should be comin' through anytime, if I remembered my rounds correctly.

I waited.

And waited.

No one came.

What was the holdup? *I'm getting hungry over here, so if you don't mind, come in, ask me if I've farted, and give me some breakfast.* Still no one showed. I looked over at Matt, who'd at some point acquired a chair-bed overnight, sleeping soundly.

Finally, they did show up, but it wasn't the occurrences in my lower digestive tract that concerned them this time; rather a lack of activity in the parathyroid department. "Your parathyroid levels aren't bouncing back like we expected them to," one of them said. Dr. Rogers was not to be seen. Where was he? I missed Dr. Wolff. In the end, they decided to keep doing draws every four hours, and I got to have an extra cup of fruit-flavored Tums out of the deal. That was something.

Finally, I was able to lose the pneumatic leg warmers after I took a few laps around the ward. I was determined to stay up and about. I needed a shower and wondered how I would do it with my neck sliced in half.

The nurse disconnected me from my drip and gave me some baby shampoo, a bar of soap, a comb, toothbrush, and toothpaste. As she started to walk out the door, I stopped her. "Hey, I need this line heparinized." She looked at me like I was insane and said no. I looked at *her* like she'd skipped the remedial nursing class. "But the line will *clot* if you don't flush it with heparin."

Then she spoke to me very slowly as though I were the thick one. "We don't flush with heparin without doctor's orders," she said simply. What? *Since when?* But I kept quiet. I was trying to be nicer than I'd been in the last few weeks. I was thinking, though, *You know, I'm not a first timer. I'm old hat at all this stuff, and I know that if you don't want to have IV therapy come up here and start a new line you gotta hep-lock this one!* I muttered "Fine" and proceeded to my shower. I learned quickly, through trial and error, that I had to support the weight of my head with one hand while I washed my hair with the other hand to avoid screaming pain in the neck region. My hair was thick and crunchy from the iodine wash, as though I'd dumped a bottle of hairspray on myself. It took three shampoos to get it all out. Then I brushed my teeth, combed my hair (again taking care to support my head with my hand), and put on a new gown. It felt good to be clean. As I walked back to my newly made bed, I remembered the old days having one tub, one shower, and two toilets for the entire ward, and I thanked God that these rooms now had their own bathrooms. When I got back into bed, I noticed a thin line of blood creeping through the clear tube on the IV. It was already clotting. Crap. If I had to get another IV just because one nurse wouldn't flush my line, I wasn't even going to try and be polite about it.

Finally, discharge orders came that evening around five, after the docs had realized there'd been an error in the lab work and my calcium levels were totally fine. I finally got to go home to spend my senior year spring break convalescing. Fun.

As the day had worn on, the plastic dressing over my throat was getting itchier and itchier. The residents, on their evening rounds, said it would come off on its own in a week or so, but they could take it off if I wanted. *No way,* I thought. *Not unless you're putting me to sleep again.* It was bad enough having doctors grab and push on your throat all the time. Nobody was getting near the throat that they'd just operated on to peel away sticky plastic. It was that stiff plastic dressing, too. The kind that looks embossed with a cross-hatch pattern. No sir.

I sighed. Was it really too much to ask to just finish college off like a normal kid and not have to think about surgeries or itchy dressings or heparin locks?

Thirty-six hours later, it was so uncomfortable I couldn't stand it anymore. I tried to take it off myself but was too psyched out. It pulled on the tiny hairs on my skin and made my eyes water with pain and anxiety. I had this irrational fear, clear as day, that I might pull it too fast and rip off some of my skin or tear the incision wide open. That, of course, led to my next irrational nightmare: tilting my head back too far and tearing the wound open, feeling my head flop down onto my shoulders. Shuddering, I tried to tell myself it wasn't logical, but once you're emotionally tied, it can be impossible to eliminate such thoughts from your mind.

Mom got the Detachol (best invention *ever*) and started to work away the corners of the dressing. I lay on my bed, sweating, eyes streaming, afraid she would hurt me. Not being able to see what was going on and not having control over it was killing me—far worse than the pain. After parts of the dressing were removed, I could feel the relief on my skin. Eventually, Mom got out a pair of scissors saying, "I'm going to trim away some of the dressing, so we don't have to get too close to your incision." I nodded at her but could barely hold still enough for her to do her work. The idea of a pair of scissors hanging around that area was too much. She tried to "tough love" some sense into me, but that only made me angry.

Finally, the blessed moment had arrived. I looked at myself in the mirror. A small, crude oval remained where the large square had been, thanks to Mom's scissors. The skin that had been under it was red and inflamed, such that my pink leathery bib looked normal in comparison. It felt luxurious to let that skin breathe again. I delicately rubbed the area with aloe in hopes of hastening the healing process, and slept marvelously that night.

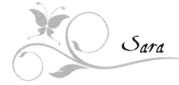

One of Lindsey's friends, Carly, decided to have a party for her treatments. She called it the "Hey Hey, Ho Ho, This Thyroid Cancer's Got to Go" party. Again, I didn't quite know what to think about being so glib about something so serious. Instead of that whispered, "Oh, no, she's got cancer *" that I was so used to, it was more like, "This sucks. LET'S PARTY!" It was so cool to be able to go to this party and have fun with it all. I was so appreciative of Carly for being there during those times. Their personalities were very similar, and that's what Lindsey needed. Someone who would be sarcastic and laugh and just call it what it was. All I wanted to do was cry in the corner all the time, and that's probably not what she needed at all.*

After a week of convalescence, I went with Matt to Seattle before returning to Spokane and school. My new endocrinologist had given me meds to bring my thyroid levels back to normal quickly, and I was feeling pretty good. Dr. Rogers had ordered me to stand up straight, adding, "It's not like you're going to tear open your stitches," which was all I needed to hear. I did exercises, trying to get my range of motion back. My throat felt hard, completely unyielding. As hard as a wood floor. Had it always been like that? I thought it hadn't. Rogers explained it was part of the healing process, and that it would soften up in time.

The next phase in treatment would be nuclear medicine. Endocrinology explained that there would be no chemo or radiation, and certainly no bone marrow transplant. I was stunned. Who'd ever heard of cancer treatment without chemo? I'd spent so much time over the past weeks and months agonizing over what it would be like to do it all again, and seriously considering declining treatment. Although I didn't tell anyone that because I knew they'd all wig out. But this process was totally different. And fascinating. Instead of chemo, they would give me a certain amount of the iodine isotope I-131, and I would remain in isolation until I'd excreted the nuclear material. Because the thyroid is the only organ in the body that uses iodine, it and only it would suck up the radiation and kill itself. There was hardly any tissue to kill, either—just the little bits still attached to the parathyroids (and occasionally thyroid tissue can grow in other parts of the body, like behind the sternum). So, I wouldn't get sick, lose my hair, or have myelosuppression. Though I was instructed not to spend time around small pets, old people, or pregnant women for a week or so.

In preparation for the I-131 treatment, I had to stop taking my meds and undergo a diet that slowly robbed my body of iodine, so what tissue was left would be good and hungry. Thus, I was forced to drop all foods that had red dye #30 in them, seafood, turkey, condiments, potatoes, breads, chocolate, and dairy. I could eat most raw fruits and vegetables, beef and, surprisingly, have as much alcohol as I wanted, malt or hard. I subsisted on T-Bone steaks with sautéed onions and mushrooms, fruit, and water for the most part. It got old, though, living in a house where my roommates got to eat pizza, cereal, and Taco Bell whenever they wanted.

As I went on and my thyroid levels dipped, I became slow. I took a lot of naps, and at work I had problems focusing on what was going on. On more than one occasion, I sat at the audio board going through rote motions while essentially all other senses dozed, and I would gradually wake up to:

"Hey, Lindsey?" Pause.

"Lindsey." Another pause.

"Yo, Lindsey!"

"What?" as I turned dopily toward the director.

"When are we back from commercial?"

"Oh…thirty seconds."

The other thing I noticed with all this flux in medications, and suddenly being unable to produce my own thyroid hormones, was rage. A problem in one system in the body will have a trickle-down effect on the others, even if minutely. This was not a minute problem, however. When I wasn't dozing, I was responding to the smallest inconveniences with disproportionally inappropriate, uncontrollable, all-out rage. For instance, I had recently bought a tapeless answering machine for the house from Target. I set it up, saw that it worked, and threw the boxes out. Within two weeks it failed, spewing out distorted digital garble rather than our missed calls. I called the store and explained the situation that the boxes and receipts were gone, but because this product malfunctioning so badly, would they take it back? They said yes. They could trace the transaction through the Visa I'd used. I found myself standing at the Customer Service counter arguing with a manager about this conversation. The end result was no, they *couldn't* trace it through my Visa (they didn't know how I'd come up with that idea). And they *wouldn't* take it back without the boxes. What could I—*should* I—have done? Been irate. Filed a complaint. Then chocked it up to a $30 loss and move on. What *did* I do? I yelled at the employees, accusing them of wasting my time and lying to their customers. I postulated that I would boycott Target from now on. Then I grabbed the answering machine by its cord and dragged it out of the store and into the parking lot where I proceeded to beat the shit out of it on the asphalt before flinging it into the trash, stomping off to my car, and peeling out for home.

This kind of thing happened with increasing frequency during and after the whole treatment process. I couldn't control it. It was almost like I was watching myself act this way from outside my own body. Part of my brain could stand back and mutter, *This is really inappropriate. You need to mellow out.* Then the other, more powerful part of my brain would counter, *Shut up! I do what I want! Nobody controls me!* Balancing out hormones is not a quick process, either. It took the better part of a year to get my levels at a place that were comfortable for me, and even longer to work past the emotional trauma of the winter of 2002 (what I blithely referred to as The Winter of My Discontent). However, thyroid hormone demands can be dynamic, and even today the first clue I get that my meds are too low or too high—before I have sleeping problems or cold intolerance or sweats—is an inappropriate rage response. It takes a lot of mental work to temper that.

Finally, the day arrived when I found myself back at OHSU in the Nuclear Medicine department. Much to my surprise and gratitude, it had moved since last I'd been there, and now actually looked like a modern department. They prepared me for what would happen during the nuclear treatment. I would take the pill containing the isotope, and they would actually take a reading on me with a Geiger counter. Then, they'd shut the door and I wouldn't be allowed out until my levels were down to normal again. They'd read me with the Geiger counter every twenty-four hours. The nurse would wear a beeper that would warn her when to leave the room. The room would be covered in plastic, because the oils in my skin would also put out radiation. My food would be served on disposable plates and trays. I could be there overnight, or I could be there for a week, depending on dose.

In order to determine what dose I should get, they needed to do a tracer test. That day, they gave me a pill that had five millicuries of I-131 in it. Twenty-four hours later, I returned for a special scan that would detect the presence of the substance in my body and show them where it had been absorbed. That was where things got scary.

I showed up for the scan, which was pretty easy. Easier than any CT scan I'd done. I just sat there, very still, and breathed normally. When it was done—and it took a long time—I was sent to the waiting room. Mom and I waited for quite a while before the guy came to get us. He took us to a back room—never a good sign—to talk with some more people. I could see my scans were on the computer behind him. He started to explain them.

"Anything that's green shows uptake of the isotope." I looked. I had a bright green spot in my throat, some in my stomach and very little on my arms. "Now," he continued, "the thyroid area is very bright, which is fine, and there usually is some uptake in the lining of the stomach, which there is, just because of digestion, and your limbs should be black, which they almost are." I looked at the hazy green silhouette of my body, wondering what the problem was. "The problem is here," he pointed to my lungs. "There should be no uptake there because it's all airspace. The lungs shouldn't absorb anything." My lungs were clearly defined in electric green clouds. *Oh, God.*

Mom and I stood there in the hallway. I stared open mouthed at the screen. At my lungs. *What the hell?* I was tired of this roller coaster: You have cancer. But it's not the bad kind. But we're doing surgery. But don't worry because we're not doing chemo. But now you're lungs are green. We're all quite worried about that. I didn't even know how to respond. Again, the myriad of emotions and memories pulsed through my brain. Were my lungs full of tumors again? Would I need a lung transplant? God, when would this all just *stop*?

"Since we're not quite sure what's going on there, we want to give you another twenty-four hours. How much water do you drink?" one guy asked me.

I shrugged. "I don't know. I drink when I'm thirsty."

"OK, well, drink as much water as possible. There's a chance this just hasn't managed to move through yet."

The ride home was silent, apprehensive. I pounded as much water as I could stomach that night—never an easy or pleasant task—and slept fitfully awaiting the next scan.

Twenty-four hours later I found myself again on the table for the chest portion of the nuclear scan. I waited for the test to complete, anxiously anticipating the results. What if my lungs were full of tumors? How could that be possible? Wouldn't Dr. Wolff have caught it already? It wasn't like I didn't go to the doctor like four times a year just for routine checkups. I hadn't noticed any exceptional breathing problems. I was working out fairly regularly without any incident. God, if I had tumors in my lungs again, they'd probably scratch the nuclear treatment and ship me off to the BMT unit straight away.

Mom and I sat in silence, waiting for the scan to be read. Finally, the pack of doctors who had seen me yesterday came out. One of them said, "The field looks clear, so it was probably just a matter of needing some extra time to flush things out." I heaved a sigh of relief, feeling the ton of bricks being lifted from my chest—or maybe it was my imaginary tumors disappearing. He continued, "So, we'll see you day after tomorrow for the actual treatment."

"What's the dose?" I asked.

"We don't know for sure yet, but based on the amount of uptake we see in the field, probably one of the lowest doses ever." I was satisfied with that. So I'd probably only be in isolation for a few days instead of the week that I was expecting.

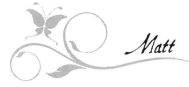

Matt

I had some make-up work to do because of how upset Lindsey was about me not being there when she was diagnosed. I don't think it was so much about me being in Arizona when she was going through this; it was that she couldn't get a hold of me when the cancer-call came in.

And then it all went exactly as planned. The doctors said that treatment wasn't an invasive procedure, there was little chance of it spreading, and everything turned out fine, just as expected.

Sara

When we found out how they were going to treat it, I thought that was actually pretty cool. Radioactive isotopes! That seemed a lot better than all the typical treatments you read about. Especially compared to what they'd done to her before. Totally cool.

The next morning, we arrived at OHSU and reported to the eighth floor. The nurses directed me to a private room in the back of the ward, the door to which was decorated with a large yellow and purple biohazard sign. The guys from nuclear medicine met us in the room and instructed me to put my clothes in a bag in the closet and not touch them until discharged. I was wearing the old staple: white and blue gown emblazoned with "OHSU" and gray treaded socks. The counters, bed rails, faucets, sinks, doorknobs, telephone, and walls were wrapped in either thick paper or plastic wrap. There was an enormous Rubbermaid garbage can in the room labeled with the same yellow and purple sign that graced the door.

"Everything except you and your clothes that comes in here, stays in here," said the nuclear medicine guy as he pointed to the garbage can. "Your nurse wears a meter, and can only be in here for a few minutes at a time. You will be emitting radiation, so do not flush the toilet or take a shower. We don't want that radiation flowing through the pipes of the hospital and exposing other patients. All the stuff in this room is wrapped because the oils in your skin will also emit radiation."

I was stunned and amazed. We'd only invented nuclear technology fifty years ago, and the instructions they were giving me were probably still not everything there is to know about radiation. They explained that my salivary glands could take up some of the radiation, and that I needed to drink lots of water and suck on hard candy to keep the glands clear.

After all the questions were answered, he whipped out a large gray canister. He unscrewed the lid and poured the contents into a paper cup. I looked in. A small pill was in there. It was smaller, even, than the old Septra antibiotics I used to take. Actually, it was very anticlimactic.

"That's 101 millicuries," he said. I had to follow specific instructions to take it. First, take a drink of water, then by only touching the paper cup it was in, swallow the pill, then take another drink of water. Then, show them that I'd actually swallowed the pill. They pointed a Geiger meter at me and left the room. They closed the door and measured the radiation from outside the room, and I was alone.

Jeanna had brought me two paper grocery bags full of stuff. She said she'd wrapped up a bunch of corny surprises so I wouldn't get bored. I thought about tearing into them right away, to see what was up, but remembered I might have to last seventy-two hours in here. Watch, they'd come get me in 3 days and I would be dead of boredom. I left the grocery bags for later. In the meantime, I took my crayons that I'd brought and started to draw all over the paper that covered the room.

Surprisingly, I was only in there for twenty-four hours—practically a new record—and I entertained myself by watching TV with my plastic-wrapped remote, talking on the plastic-wrapped phone, blowing bubbles, and perfecting my crayon-and-paper magnum opus.

Dinner was uneventful: a plastic, disposable tray laden with paper and Styrofoam products boasting lame, sodium-free, low-iodine foods. I couldn't wait for this diet to be over. When I got out of here, I wanted a hefty slab of pepperoni from Pizza Schmizza with a Coke and an ice cream sundae for dessert. Every food I'd been denied for the last three weeks all rolled into one meal. Almost every food. I guess I'd have to have a big fat shrimp cocktail for an appetizer.

In the morning, the guy from nuclear medicine came again with his Geiger counter. He pointed it at me from the doorway, and said in a surprised tone, "Well, your levels are pretty low. I think you'll be out of here tonight. I'll come back around four for another reading." I called Mom so she could order a pizza and stock up on Coke and ice cream for that night. The day couldn't pass fast enough. I tore through the all the toys and games Jeanna had sent: mini Etch-a-sketch, fake jewelry, travel games, penny whistles, and that kind of thing. It helped pass two hours.

Then the blessed moment arrived.

I put my real clothes on and left the hospital with instructions to stay away from small animals, children, old people, and pregnant women for the next week or so. I wasn't allowed near Sandy Dunes. But as I sat by myself on one end of the breakfast bar, I gorged on pizza, Coke, and ice cream that night with Mom, Dad, and Travis. It was as though I'd never tasted it before. I was so happy.

PART THREE:

Reconstruction

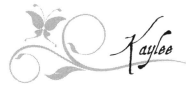
Kaylee

There's this population of people in my life–parents, patients, siblings–that when I see them, even years later, I'm overwhelmed. We shared this incredible experience together. I ran into a sibling at the mall a year ago or so. She came up and hugged me and got all teary, and I got all teary. I took care of her brother when he was dying. And a lot of times, years later, parents will still call us with a problem, and new nurses try to make them call a primary care doctor instead. They don't understand the dynamic of trust with these oncologists. It's a lifelong bond.

Because I'd finished all of my coursework before leaving Gonzaga for treatment, I returned to Spokane with just enough time to finish the packing I'd started and walk at graduation. I was the only one in my house who didn't have any finals. I spent my days sleeping in and taking the meds that would bring my metabolism back up to speed. The meds that I would take for the rest of my life—a thought that was more depressing every day. The idea of taking off on a whim for a trip somewhere for any length of time was out of the question. I would always have to round up my pharmacopeia first and make sure I had enough. Lame.

When graduation day came, I donned the oddly expensive but clearly cheap polyester blue gown and mortarboard, stole, hood, and the cords from my numerous honor societies: gold for Magna Cum Laude, red and white for Lambda Pi Eta, blue and yellow for Psi Chi, and a gold medallion on a burgundy ribbon for Alpha Sigma Nu. I received baccalaureates in psychology and broadcast communications. Not exactly what the four-year plan was originally, but it was good enough for me. For now. Next thing I knew, the party was over, the truck was loaded, and I drove the old green Subaru West on I-90, gleefully watching the Spokane skyline recede in the rearview mirror. That chapter was over. No more TV news. No more meth heads wandering through my neighborhood. No more Gonzaga. I was ready for a vacation and some new adventures.

However, my vacation ended up going much longer than I anticipated. I aimed to take three months off and actively search for my job for a month. I figured it might take couple of months to get one.

I had no idea what I was in for.

I wanted a job in Portland. Matt was still in Seattle, but I didn't want to move up there for anything. Rule number one had always been to never follow a man anywhere. He could follow me if he wanted. Seattle was huge, had too many people on the road, and was too expensive (that's my father talking). The unspoken reason, of course, was that I didn't want to leave my "home." That is, OHSU and Dr. Wolff. I couldn't stand the idea of finding myself in a cancer crisis without him within arm's reach again.

That summer I split my time between Portland and Seattle with Matt, and explored opportunities with American Cancer Society. I attended Camp UKANDU, this time heading up the music department. Afterward, I managed the production of the Camp UKANDU CD–a collection of the most popular camp songs to be given out to all of the campers every year. I even got some of the actual campers into the act. As I started actively looking for jobs, I found that the task would be far more difficult than I ever imagined. Matt was firmly planted in Seattle, and I resented him for it. But things deteriorated to a point where I had to make a decision: I could either break up with him, or suck it up and move.

On principle, I should break up with him.

However, if I was going to really give it my best, then I should move. But if I moved, my chances of being self-reliant were even less, and in fact, Matt would have to support me until I could snag a job, because I was having zero luck finding one from here. Besides, what if I moved and still resented him? This was all so complicated. I was scared.

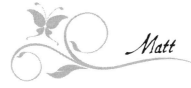

Matt

When she told me she didn't ever want kids, I thought, Oh, that's just her adolescence talking. Nobody wants to have children when they're twenty years old. *Once I learned about the difficulty associated with having kids when you only have one kidney, I understood better. But I was still in denial. So what? Sure it's a high-risk pregnancy, but a lot of people do it. So it's not that big of an obstacle if you want to have kids.*

But she didn't.

The National Wilms Tumor Study Group Data and Statistical Center is located at the Fred Hutchinson Cancer Research Center in Seattle. I contacted them and received a complete copy of my medical records. I received published articles regarding late effects studies and treatment protocol studies—including the one I participated in. My big interest was in sterility. I knew that my radiation fields had encompassed the lower abdomen, which meant that my ovaries and uterus had more than likely been irradiated. Plus, I'd received both actinomycin D and cyclophosphamide, agents that have been known to cause sterility in certain doses. That, coupled with the fact that I stopped ovulating at eighteen–even after taking the normally prescribed oral contraceptives for two years it still hadn't resolved–was leading me to believe I might be sterile.

Dr. Wolff had given me a copy of *Childhood Cancer Survivors: A Practical Guide to Your Future.* It detailed different types of cancers, leukemias, and treatments that children endure, and helped guide us survivors into what that meant for the rest of our lives, including impacts on medical insurance, relationships, and late-effects. Sterility was definitely a side effect to some treatments–more common when certain chemos were combined with radiation to the abdomen and pelvis. I picked the brains of every physician on my team. Dr. Wolff couldn't tell me for sure, so he suggested I consult with OB/GYN at OHSU. They said that there was no reliable way to tell for sure until I tried having children, and if I wasn't able, then there were all sorts of treatments I could explore to enhance the chance of conception. That idea sickened me. I knew what was involved in fertility treatments, and it wasn't non-invasive. Endocrinology posited much the same. They suggested that it's possible I'd suffered primary ovarian failure, but it would be almost impossible to know for sure until the day arrived that I wanted to try conceiving. The idea of being sterile didn't bother me. I just wanted to know so that I could plan contraception.

I thought back to the day almost ten years before when Dr. Stein said I could well be sterile and that I could take the pill, juggling so that I did get my periods, or juggling it so that I wouldn't. I certainly wasn't distraught. I hadn't wanted kids since we'd had that conversation with Dr. Stein in the first place, and the very idea of pregnancy was nauseating: the edema, the stretch marks, the nausea, the vomiting, the weight gain, the gestational hypertension and diabetes, the hemorrhoids, and the idea that something was growing in there. That didn't even encompass all the bad things that could happen, such as preeclampsia. Not to mention even the remotest possibility that any progeny could inherit my cancer genes. *No, thank you.* In my mind, who could ever, in good conscience, deliberately create an innocent knowing it stood a risk of suffering debilitating disease? I could not live with the idea of any child of mine enduring what I endured. I knew too well what it was like.

It was a problem for Matt, though. He seemed convinced I was going through a phase and I'd grow out of it eventually "as soon as [my] biological clock starts ticking." I found this offensive and told him that he needed to seriously reevaluate his situation, and if he absolutely, hands-down, had to have biological kids in his life, then he needed to move on. I agreed to be open to the possibility, but I wasn't making any promises. I'd much sooner adopt a child who is alone on this earth than create more mouths for the planet to feed. I cannot see a quantifiable difference anyway. Commit social justice and avoid pregnancy, or tacitly approve children who are hungry and alone, with no hope for success in life, *and* have to endure pregnancy? Whatever. The answer seemed pretty crystal to me. If he wanted kids so bad, then let *him* be pregnant!

Before ever moving to Seattle I gave him an ultimatum: figure it out and call me back. He called the next night and said that our relationship was more important to him than the potential of children. I hoped he was being honest with himself.

Sterility and my hormonal imbalances continued to occupy my mind. I wondered if I should stop taking the pill to see if my body had corrected itself yet, worrying that it hadn't, and the effects I would have to feel. These worries were usurped by much bigger ones in the spring of 2003.

Shortly after Matt asked me to marry him, I started having problems breathing—or so it seemed. I found myself sitting around the apartment or at work, doing nothing in particular, and suddenly my pulse would skyrocket to 115 and I felt I couldn't get any air. At first, I thought it must be an anxiety attack. I tried to think rationally through these attacks, to find the source for my worries, and I couldn't find any triggers or anything wrong except that it felt like the oxygen wasn't passing through my lungs. I mentioned the symptoms to Matt and Mom, and they both insisted that I was just worried about something. Worried about *what?*

"I used to have anxiety attacks all the time when I was your age. That's probably what you're going through," Mom advised. She continued to tell me how she'd overcome it and how I could get through the attacks. I didn't believe that. I'd studied anxiety and panic disorders a little in school, and I really didn't think that's what I'd been experiencing. It didn't quite fit. I'd been in touch with Endocrinology about it, and they thought maybe my thyroid dose was too high, but when the blood test came back, I was in the normal range. She entertained the idea that I could have some late effects from radiation or something.

"If it happens again, call me," she ordered. I waited. Time passed.

Finally, on Easter Sunday, Matt and I went to Mass with his mother. During the Liturgy of the Eucharist, as I knelt in the pew, reading the *Missal,* I had the worst attack yet. I couldn't breathe. My heart was racing. I looked around. God, I couldn't breathe! I took my pulse. It was over one hundred. I was surrounded by people, with no way to escape from the stuffy church, wedged between Matt and his mom. I choked back tears that threatened to burst over my lids and betray what I was going through to all these strangers. I held them back, stuffing the hot sensation back down my throat, focused on forcing myself to take long, deep (but unproductive) breaths, and waited for Mass to conclude. The priests droned on. I didn't hear a word. Fifteen minutes later, we walked out into the sunshine, and the fresh air didn't help. After taking his mother home, Matt and I walked into our apartment and he started gathering up his gear to go to work—he shot for the news department on Sundays.

I picked up the phone to page my endocrinologist. I was officially panicked, now. *This* was panic.

"Who are you calling?" Matt asked.

"Dr. Takemoto," I retorted.

"Why?"

"Because I had another one of those attacks in church. It was really bad."

"Really? I didn't notice anything was wrong."

"Well, what was I supposed to do? I couldn't get out and leave, and it's so *embarrassing*. So I just tried to stay calm. I don't know what's happening!" I could feel that if this conversation went on, I would lose it. What was wrong with me? Everything was supposed to be fine now. *There is no more cancer. I'm supposed to be having a completely normal life.* Dr. Takemoto wasn't available, but there was another endocrinologist on call. I didn't see how this woman would help me, but I didn't have anywhere else to go. Even Dr. Wolff wouldn't be able to help me with this one. I agreed, and the switchboard operator took my number and said she'd have the doctor on call give me a ring.

Matt waited with me for the return call before leaving for work. When the doctor finally called, I started to describe my symptoms, and while I was listing off my problems, I saw everything so lucidly, so terrifyingly. I had no idea what was wrong with me. I couldn't fix it. I couldn't cope through it. It kept happening. I started to hitch my breath, feeling the tears right behind it. I couldn't talk. Matt took the phone from me.

"Hi," he said into the phone. "She's really scared right now, I think. She doesn't know why this is happening, and it keeps happening." The doc asked about my medications, my TSH levels, and whether I'd had any heart problems before or had a history of anxiety. We told her that I'd had chest radiation and been treated with cyclophosphamide and Adriamycin. She didn't have any suggestions for me, and said she'd relay all this information to Dr. Takemoto the next day.

"Just stay home and keep it low for the day. Relax."

I curled up on the bed and sobbed into the pillow. Matt sat next to me, rubbing my back comforting me.

"I don't know what's wrong!" I shrieked into the pillow.

"I'm staying home from work today to be with you," Matt said as he dialed the newsroom. I rolled over and looked out the window at the Puget Sound and the jagged snow peaked Olympic Mountains fading on the horizon. I guess if I had to feel this crummy, at least Matt would be with me for the day. He called in sick and then called Dominoes. "You hungry? Let's get a pizza, OK?" I nodded. I was hungry. It was Easter Sunday—*the highest feast day on the Catholic calendar, and we're ordering a pizza*, I thought wryly.

When I finally talked to Dr. Takemoto again, she was concerned for my heart and arranged an appointment with a colleague in cardiology. I drove down to OHSU in late May to see Dr. Gladstone. When he walked in, I was struck dumb by how much he looked like actor Henry Gibson, who played Dr. Klopek in that 80s movie *The Burbs*. Of course, that's all I could think about during the whole visit. I wanted to ask him, *do you* drive *your garbage cans to the curb, Dr. Gladstone? Do you have a creepy furnace in your basement?* He did a physical and asked a few questions like "Does exercise induce these attacks?" and "Have you been keeping track of how high your pulse goes?" I learned that a pulse up to 120 bpm was still considered normal. He didn't suspect anything was seriously wrong but thought some follow-up work would be necessary, considering I'd had radiation to the chest and been treated with both anthracyclines and cyclophosphamide. Dr. Wolff agreed that I should have some baseline cardiology work done anyway because of my treatment history. *This stuff never ends.* Even when the cancer is *over*, it's not over.

"Lindsey, tell me about your life. What do you do? What's been happening the last year or so?" I was surprised. I told him I'd been diagnosed with cancer, graduated from college, been unemployed, gotten engaged, and moved away from my family in the last year. He nodded, making notes in my chart. "Do you work?" he wondered.

"Yeah. I work at the CBS affiliate in Seattle."

His raised eyebrows suggested he'd seen the light. "And how would you describe your work environment?"

I actually hated my work environment. I mean, it was better than KXLY, but it was still the same old crap. I made ten dollars an hour and wasn't allowed more than twenty-five hours a week. I did the grunt job that no one else in the newsroom quite understood or appreciated, and when I couldn't do my job because the writers and reporters weren't doing theirs, I was the one who got in trouble with the anchors or management. At KXLY I would get called into the news director's aquarium office and he would scream red-faced at me. KIRO was considerably quieter but not all that different. People were always getting mad over ratings numbers that no one understood. It seemed so dumb to me. "It's hectic," I finally answered. "Low pay, split shifts, low glass ceiling." I shrugged at him.

He stopped writing and looked me in the eye. "You've got a lot on your plate. You've had four major life-changing events happen in the last year, and since you're getting married, you've got one more major life event on the way within the next four months. I'm going to write you a prescription for Toprol, which is a beta-blocker. It prevents adrenaline from maxing out your heart, which is what I suspect is happening. I think you're on adrenaline over-load." I nodded. That made sense to me. He continued, "I'm giving you the smallest dose, and if you think that's too big, then break the pill in half. It should help bring things down for you." He handed me the script. "Do you meditate? Do yoga?" he asked.

"I have in the past."

"I also want you to be doing yoga or meditation or tai chi. Something that can help you diffuse everything around you and bring your adrenaline levels down." I agreed. I'd always wanted to do yoga anyway. It might be fun. He finished by saying, "Then we're going to do an echo to see where you are after all the treatments you had all those years ago."

So it sounded like the top heart doc thought I had anxiety, too. Well, it wasn't the first time Linda might have been right about something. I didn't *feel* like I "had anxiety," but then again, I guess I didn't know exactly what it's supposed to feel like. It must feel like...me.

Echo tests are all right. You got to lie in a dark room and doze, while they pushed the stylus around on your chest and clicked on a keyboard, marking images I never understood how anyone could read. Painless.

To make a long story short, my heart was fine. There was some debate about whether or not there was a "density" in one of the valves. They resolved this by doing a TEE—transesophageal echo—that would give them a clearer picture. For once in my life, it was hard to hear the good news that nothing was wrong. I was instructed to see cardiology and have an echo once every year just for the standard follow-up care. In the meantime, I loved the beta-blockers. I was down to a resting pulse of sixty-five or so. A first! I hadn't felt this comfortable in a very long time.

The small bout with the heart issue initiated thoughts on my kidney. The nephrologist I had seen years before had said I'd never need a GFR again. I wondered about that. I wanted to make sure that I was doing everything I could to protect my kidney. I didn't ever want to be on a transplant list. Maybe I should talk to another nephrologist. Or maybe I should just quit worrying about it and trust his professional judgment. It was things like this that made my pulse shoot through the roof—right?

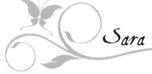

Matt

I think as the years have gone by, she has been able to distance herself from the bad thoughts and memories associated with cancer. She is better at coping with all of it now. It's made me grow up a lot, too. I've learned a lot about relationships, and I know more about cancer now than I ever dreamed of. It was my first encounter with the disease, and it opened my eyes.

Sara

She has to go have her checkup tests done every once in awhile, and I'm prepared for those to not to come back all right someday. And I'm also prepared to be on a plane the next morning and go sit in a corner and cry with her. It's funny. I want to be a supportive friend, but really, I think I'd also kind of need her *to support* me, *too, because she's the steely one.*

It was time to acknowledge that I was now in the long-term follow up phase. I had to be careful about but not obsessed with the idea of cancer returning, so I needed to organize and keep better track of my follow-up. I was glad that the Seattle Cancer Care Alliance and the National Wilms Tumor Study Group were right there to oversee everything. They kept track of what tests had to be done during which year (i.e., mammograms, blood tests, MRIs, colonoscopies, urine samples, echos, etc.) and how often those should be repeated. If that had all been up to me, I would've been completely overwhelmed and just quit. They also referred me to specific specialists who were familiar with peds cancer long term follow up—not necessarily an easy thing to come by.

They send me newsletters every so often detailing new research findings about long term side effects. Over time, it has become easier to accept this phase and resume a "normal" life. It's not easy because everyone around me pretty much eats, drinks, and does whatever they want. I have to constantly redouble my efforts to maintain my leftover bits. For the kidney, it's a low sodium, low fat, low protein, low phosphorus, and low potassium diet. This includes restricting myself to one cup of coffee a day and restricting alcohol to just once or twice a month. It's not easy at all, because I've morphed into a foodie and I'm always looking for my next taste adventure, which doesn't often mesh all that well with the restricted diet. For the lung, I really have to keep up on the exercise or else I get winded and wheezy pretty easily. I can't forget a healthy dose of sunscreen when I go outside, since my skin cancer risk is elevated. I get my mammograms. I get screened for thyroid tumor regrowth. It's a lot of work. The nicest thing is that the more time passes, the easier it is to keep PTSD at bay, though sometimes I have nightmares or I still feel like it's January 5, 1995 all over again.

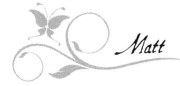

Matt

After she had gone through her difficulties in the TV industry, and she'd followed me to Seattle, she had this feeling of, "Oh, crap. What am I supposed to do?" I had this great job in Seattle, and she was in total limbo. She realized that she was supposed to be a doctor. So we decided on one fateful rainy night to go to medical school. It was a very long road to get there, but I was excited for her. I thought she would have the opportunity to fulfill a lifelong dream that she had, and I would be able to help her do it.

I am strolling down the serpentine pathway that leads to the building where my first class is. It'll be hot today, pushing one hundred degrees. The haze that is so indicative of LA hangs on the horizon, and I can see the occasional palm tree here and there. A cluster of nearby trees emits a cacophony from a flock of birds, the whoosh of sprinklers are accompanied by the smell of wet earth, and my anxiety level is about to make my head explode.

This is day one of medical college.

I can scarcely believe I am here. I'm surprised to be standing in this spot—on the outskirts of LA at a small school I'd never heard of even one year before.

When it had become clear to me in the winter of 2002 that I had gone completely off-course in college, I decided I had to go back to pre-med. I knew that if I didn't try to get into medical college, I would never be able to live with myself. I still wanted to be like Dr. Wolff. I wanted to know what he knew, speak the language that he spoke, and do the work that he did so steadfastly and professionally.

Television news was just not cutting it.

During my tenure as a news assistant, I learned that TV news puts on airs about "serving the public." Sometimes, of course, this is true—I remember working during 9/11 very clearly—but there is also a very fine line between information that serves the public and "infotainment." TV news is mostly the latter, and the industry more closely resembles the old adage, "If it bleeds, it leads" than a public service announcement. And all this work and stress and anxiety for what? Numbers. Inane numbers that don't mean anything to anyone except (maybe) the staff selling commercial spots.

Shortly after the initial thrill over having my first job in TV, I started to get the idea that I wasn't in the right place. I still loved science and medicine, but I felt like I was too far along in college to change tracks again. I tried to placate those feelings by focusing my broadcast work to emphasize medicine. Science and medicine reporting and writing, for instance. When that didn't work for me, I thought I could work in communications for a cancer association or a hospital, but try as I might, I couldn't make anything out of that, either. It occurred to me as I was preparing my resume tape that it would take me ten years to ascend to a level of reporting that would allow me to specialize in science and medicine. *I could get into and finish medical school in that time.*

Then one night at about three a.m., after I'd been on the clock for about twelve hours with a good three to five still to go, I was editing a "pedestrian vs. bus" video for the morning show. It hit me like a ton of bricks: *I'm not supposed to be doing this.* I stared at the frozen scene of a car, bathed in the blue glow of police flashers, feeling a combination of disbelief and absolute certainty at the veracity of this thought. Unbidden, my mind ran on. *I work long hours with no predictability, no weekends, no holidays. I live an on-call life. I see plenty of horrible things through this job. Why am I not in medicine?* I thought that if a news photographer and a physician were at this "pedestrian vs. bus" scene, only one of them would try to help and the other would stand back and tape it.

These feelings were compounded by feedback from some friends and family who seemed dismayed at my change to broadcasting. People would say, "I always thought you'd do something more important..." or "Why aren't you doing something good, like medicine?" Those things were hard to hear, because I worked hard in TV; I was reasonably good at what I did.

But I could not deny that broadcasting was the wrong path for me.

As I continued my stroll toward the Health Professions Center, death grip on my lunchbox, and hearing the *snick* of a digital camera behind me—Matt was snapping away a bunch of "First Day at

School" pictures to post on Facebook—I thought about the pre-med process of the last five years.

It was an exceptionally rainy night in Seattle, and Matt and I were sitting at Dick's Hamburgers ("bag o' burgers for a buck!"), when I unexpectedly and completely broke down. Barely able to coherently form sentences, I wailed about how I hated my job, I hated TV, I was so stupid to bail out on pre-med. Matt listened to my tear-streaked yammering, munching on french fries all the while. After I was finished, he said, "Well, why don't you just go back to school?"

I thought about this while I hiccupped tears away. "I don't have any money to go to school," I scowled.

"OK. I'll pay for it," he said simply.

I looked darkly at him, still sniffling. "Why?"

He shrugged in response, while he dragged a fry though some ketchup. "Why not? You should be able to do what you love, and if this bothers you so much, then you should do something about it."

I was stunned. It was official now. Matt Gets It.

I was from that moment, officially a post-baccalaureate pre-medical student. The first thing I learned was that this was going to be a long and expensive process. University of Washington was overwhelmed with students and so had blocked admittance to post-baccalaureates. Moreover, all the pre-health advisors were telling me that community college wasn't going to serve me well when I was sitting before a medical admissions committee—community college just wasn't rigorous enough in their eyes. This left two options: Seattle University and Seattle Pacific University—both private and *pricey*.

For this and other reasons, I highly advise people to finish their pre-med work on their *first* pass through college.

The result was three years of work at four different schools, trying to cobble together the right credits for the most efficient price possible, in the right period of time. For cost reasons, I decided to try to do my lower division coursework at community colleges, while doing the organic chemistry and calculus at Seattle University—home of my good pals, the Jesuits.

Pre-medical studies are an exercise in absolute perfection. Medical school matriculants always have incredibly high GPAs, high MCAT scores, and are generally the most generous, amazing superhero volunteers you've ever seen. They are brilliantly articulate and knowledgeable in many areas of politics and research. On top of all that, a lot of them are *pretty*. It's a very intimidating crowd to run with.

Pre-med is also an incredible gamble, I found out. In the U.S. there are some forty thousand applicants every year for the seventeen thousand available seats in MD schools. The ratios are similar for the Doctor of Osteopathic Medicine (DO) schools–physicians who are functionally and legally equivalent to MDs with additional training in musculoskeletal manual medicine. I was scared that if I couldn't get in to a professional school, this financial gamble would be all for naught—pre-med coursework is not equivalent to a new degree and is not conducive to a built-in backup plan.

In short, I came out all right in the end. My GPA ended up right where it should have. My MCAT scores were about two points lower than I wanted. I began the process of applying to medical schools.

The first attempt was a bust.

I applied to nineteen MD schools in June 2007 (not yet knowing a thing about what a DO was). I received interview invitations at Georgetown University and University of Washington. Both of those interview experiences were beyond hard core and left me feeling like a total jackass about the paths I had taken in life, and even made my cancer experiences seem stupid. While I was glad to be out of TV, I felt it had been useful to me. I was glad that I was choosing professional school after having worked in the real world. I knew it was right. Plus, I felt that my experience as a chronic patient would be useful to have as a physician, so I might provide a better care experience to my patients. No one at the universities seemed to agree. I received no acceptances or wait-lists. Come April 2008, I started to get pretty anxious. I checked the ledger for this whole pre-med adventure and felt sick when it added up to approximately twenty-seven thousand dollars.

Twenty-seven thousand dollars gone and nothing to show for it. Shortly thereafter I was at a checkup appointment with my nephrologist, and she asked me how the application process was going. I told her every gritty detail, ending with, "I don't think it matters at all that I've been through all this cancer. No one but me seems to care."

She frowned and then said, "Well, I know it's true and you know it's true, but it *does* sound pretty outrageous, all this cancer. Maybe they think you're lying."

I raised my eyebrows in surprise. Huh. Maybe they did.

The second attempt was an entirely different experience. I applied to ten MD schools and ten DO schools, feeling particularly excited about the DO schools after attending the Northwest Osteopathic Confluence in the spring. Osteopathic medicine was a whole new medical world that re-energized me with its emphasis on caring for the whole person, including using manual medicine techniques in addition to standard Western medicine. It made me wish that there had been a DO on my peds hem/onc team. I don't think it would have made a difference in the overall outcome, but I think it would have enhanced my and my family's quality of life during those years of duress. However, DOs are not all that common in the Northwest, so it's not a surprise that we don't know much about them. I felt skeptical until I mentioned to Sara that I might apply to DO schools. She gushed with excitement. "*I* have a DO! Dr. Couch! I *love* him! You should definitely be a DO." Then she added, "You know, Dr. Couch always refers to a 'couch' as a 'divan.'"

I received an interview invitation from every DO school to which I applied. These interview experiences were wildly different from those at MD schools. In stark contrast to the MD interviews, the DOs were very intrigued by my story and interested to know how I planned to apply this experience to my future practice. When I left my interview at Western University of Health Sciences, I walked outside into the September sunshine and felt like I'd come home.

Hardened by experience, I steeled myself for a long and grueling application season, not expecting any answers until January or later. Then, in early October, weeks before I expected any sort of reply, the Dean at Western University called me and said, "The admissions committee met yesterday and decided without hesitation to offer you a place in the class of 2013."

So here I was, relocated from the emerald hills of the Pacific Northwest to find myself in the brown and dusty suburbs of LA to attend Western University of Health Sciences and earn my Doctor of Osteopathic Medicine degree.

And I was freakin' terrified.

Ever the Queen of What Ifs, a billion possibilities and crisis scenarios flashed through my head that all came down to the same idea: what if I was too dumb to be a good doctor? I wanted to be a great doctor. I wanted to be as good as Wolff. I calmed myself by repeating my mantra: *Thousands of people before me have done this. I can do it, too* (this would become a frequent mantra that I would recite before each exam to keep myself from throwing up on the guy sitting next to me).

Then it occurred to me that medical school really wasn't *all* that different from a cancer experience. It would be exhausting. It would strain my relationships. It would be insanely expensive. In fact, one might be able to argue that it was *easier* than a cancer experience—theoretically I shouldn't be getting poisoned or sliced'n'diced.

I grabbed the handle of the door to the Health Professions Building and pulled it open, greeted by the cool rush of air conditioning. As I walked in, I thought, *Well, at least this time I can keep my hair.*

For now, at least, the cancer is over. But the memories of what I've endured will never leave me, and good or bad, I don't really want them to. But it's easy to let those memories run away with you. So it is important, I believe, to do whatever is necessary to maintain a healthy mindset—I laugh a lot. The Internet helps with that. Sometimes my sense of humor can spin out of control, though. I personally find it very funny that I'm "out of spares" now–it's the only way I can handle it. These days the only thing I can still afford to lose are my tonsils, and my lousy, good-for-nothing appendix. Glad I still have *that*.

When I can't laugh something off, though, I work through things via a journal. It helps organize my thoughts when they're frantic and running together, and satisfies my sense of prayer while recording my memories for the rest of my life. That's a pretty good deal. If I had done that during my treatments, I probably could have coped better and writing this book would have been a lot easier. The linchpin for getting through the things at which you cannot bring yourself to laugh is family and friends. Where would I have been without Holly? Without Jeanna? Without my *mom?* I cannot imagine going through these cancers without my mom. Yes, we often sparred, but she was steadfastly supportive–even when I was at my snarkiest. And my poor brother, taking a backseat to me during this whole process. Oh, the things they all endured. I cannot thank them enough.

Both cancer and medical school have a common thread: they really help you crystallize the things you like and don't like, the things you want to do and don't want to do, and whether or not your life is heading in the right direction. Now it's up to me to follow through on them. I've ticked off quite a few things from my Life's Must-Do List in recent years—this book is one of them.

The thing that surprised me most about all of these cancers was my evolving perspective on death. I would say that I was lucky in that I lived. And I came to conclude that my worst fear is not of dying. In a way, I welcome death—it will reunite me with people I have known and loved. I am not afraid of it. If I am to believe all that they taught me in Catholic school, I *shouldn't* be afraid of it. But let's be clear—I am very much afraid of suffering. My worst fear is being diagnosed again with something that would take many, many months and many, many painful processes to put into remission, or worse, all that for nothing. It takes work to remember that it's just a fear, not a likelihood.

I will not say that having had cancer as a child makes you appreciate every aspect of life and living itself, because it doesn't. It doesn't make you instantly brave. It doesn't make your life or relationships suddenly fall in to place, just because you've overcome this huge obstacle. Living with the Big C and the memories of it are far from easy, but they can be a purposeful gift—if we want them to be. I cannot conceive that God had anything to do with this. The idea of inducing suffering of this magnitude on purpose for some mysterious long term benefit (as in, "God is testing her") is a monstrous fallacy of universal proportions in my mind. I was not "meant" to get cancer three times, nor was Chris "meant" to die. Life is just always in flux. Genes rearrange. Accidents happen. *We* are the ones who can appreciate and assign importance to these awful events. I like to think that we all teach each other—certainly Chris was one of the most valuable life lessons I've ever encountered. In turn, someone will learn something pivotal from those of us who have "been there, done that." Sometimes we feel guilty for having survived, when others who were seemingly so much more deserving succumbed. That's why a survivor's life cannot be lived without purpose.

So I'll take what's left of all my giblets, and I'll live my life—as long or as short as it turns out to be—with a commitment and drive only a survivor can express.

September 2004, Seattle, WA–January 2010, Claremont, CA